SUPERFOOD

JUICES, SMOOTHIES & DRINKS

Advice and Recipes to Lose Weight, Prevent Illness, and Improve Your Emotional and Physical Health

Jason Manheim

Photography by Leo Quijano II

Skyhorse Publishing

TABLE of *Contents*

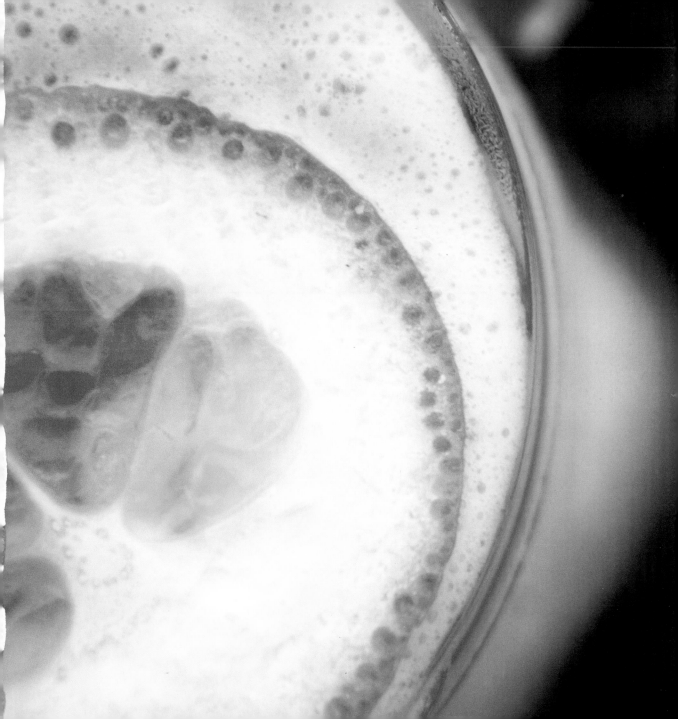

Skyhorse Publishing books may be purchased in bulk at special discounts for sales promotion, corporate gifts, fund-raising, or educational purposes. Special editions can also be created to specifications. For details, contact the Special Sales Department, Skyhorse Publishing, 307 West 36th Street, 11th Floor, New York, NY 10018 or info@skyhorsepublishing.com.

Skyhorse® and Skyhorse Publishing® are registered trademarks of Skyhorse Publishing, Inc.®, a Delaware corporation.

Visit our website at www.skyhorsepublishing.com.

10 9 8 7 6 5 4 3 2

Library of Congress Cataloging-in-Publication Data is available on file.

Cover design by Adriann Helton
Cover photo credit Leo Quijano II
Interior design by Adriann Helton
Print ISBN: 978-1-62914-592-1
Ebook ISBN: 978-1-63220-142-3
Printed in China

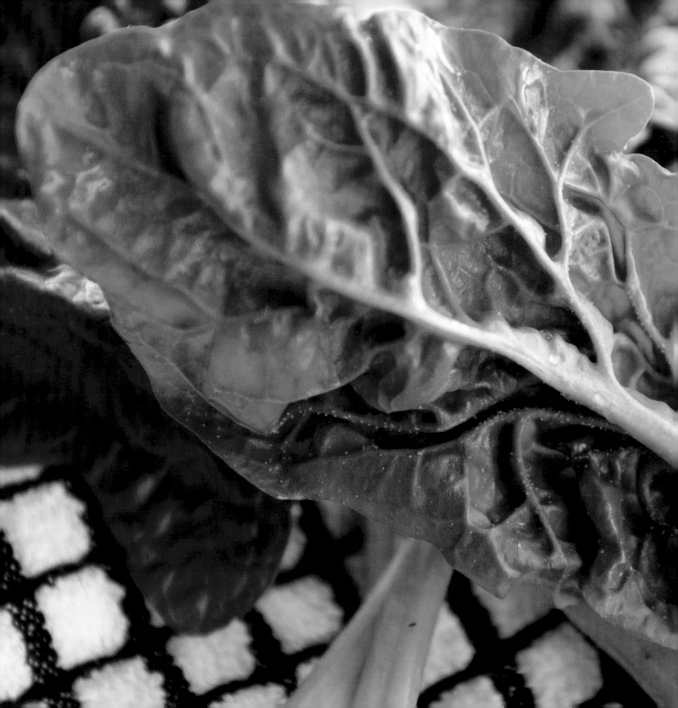

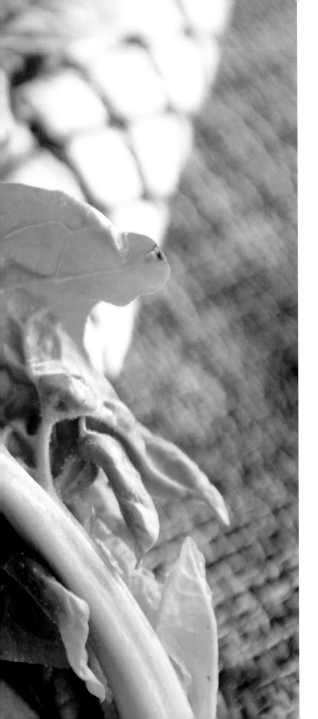

INTRODUCTION

To say superfood drinks have been a big part of my adult life would be a massive understatement. Smoothies in particular, and my trusty blender—the instrument of my wholesome libations—have altered the way I eat, feel, manage time, and ultimately approach life. A mighty claim, it may seem to the uninitiated, but a true one nonetheless. In the pages that follow, I will do my very best to equip you with the stepping stones necessary so that you may come to the same conclusion and enjoy the same feeling of ownership over at least one aspect—and a very important one at that—of your diet: simple, quick nutrition.

I never set out to *build a castle made of kale*, but like many things one becomes an authority on, it is simply an extension of an essential facet of one's daily routine—knowledge by necessity and familiarity, if you will; unavoidable.

My journey to superfood drinks started with a common modern-day gripe: *there isn't enough time in the day*. I spent the greater part of my young adult life juggling my ability to get things done with basic human functions like eating and sleeping. What a ridiculous notion it is to have to reconcile these mandatory aspects of life itself. A product of our fascination with working ourselves into the grave no doubt, but this is a book about drinks—diet and nutrition, to be precise—not meditation and balance, at least not directly.

Our motivation to eat healthier is sometimes a reaction to some sort of current malady, but also stems from our fears, or rather, our desires to avoid bad things that *may* happen in the future. These, I truly believe, are not good enough reasons. In the case of the former, it is either too late or simply damage control, and the latter is something illusory and therefore hard to hold fast. We must motivate ourselves with a more measurable reasoning. We must *eat* healthy because we want to *feel* healthy. Fantasies of avoiding illness and living *longer* should not precede the importance of living *stronger*. Everything else is a welcomed bonus.

Strength, energy, focus—these are measurable qualities that you can feel, and they should be the cornerstone of your motivation. The fact that superfood drinks provide these qualities along with a very large percentage of your daily vitamin and mineral requirements in a convenient package is what makes them so appealing.

With so many of us living fast-paced, business-oriented lives, we no longer give adequate time or thought to important activities such as food preparation and unitary sit-down meals. Instead, our meals are an afterthought, on-the-go, convenience-based choices rather than optimal selections. And because of this, our meals often lack the proper nutrition. So let me suggest the idea of replacing these quick, subpar meals with something just as quick, if not quicker, but far more healthful.

Throughout this book, you will find everything you need to make superfood drinks a foundational part of your diet. You will learn about the multitude of benefits these ingredients provide, along with a handy guide to those that are most powerful. I'll walk you through the basics of creating superfood drinks, along with templates, tools needed, how to store excess, and tips for saving money. We will explore the many diets superfood drinks lend themselves to, including detoxification, weight loss, meal replacement, and supplementation. I will then introduce you to an array of delicious recipes that can be enjoyed as-is or built upon to create the perfect drink. Recipe categories include smoothies, juices, infused waters, coffees, teas, and other drinks. To finish, I will answer some common questions and supply a list of resources and references so you may explore and expand to your heart's content.

As someone who values my time as equally as my health, my hope is that you will find the material within as helpful, manageable, and life-changing as I have. Superfood drinks: the *better* fast food. Enjoy!

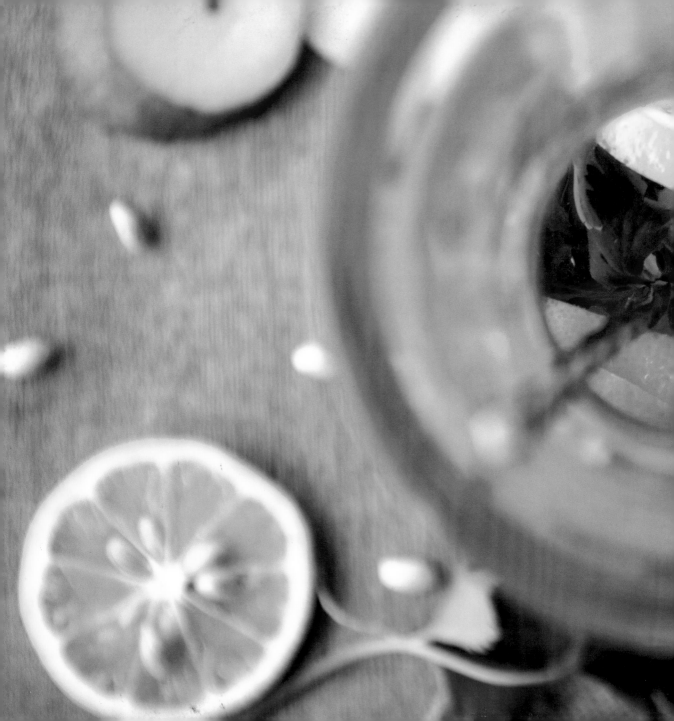

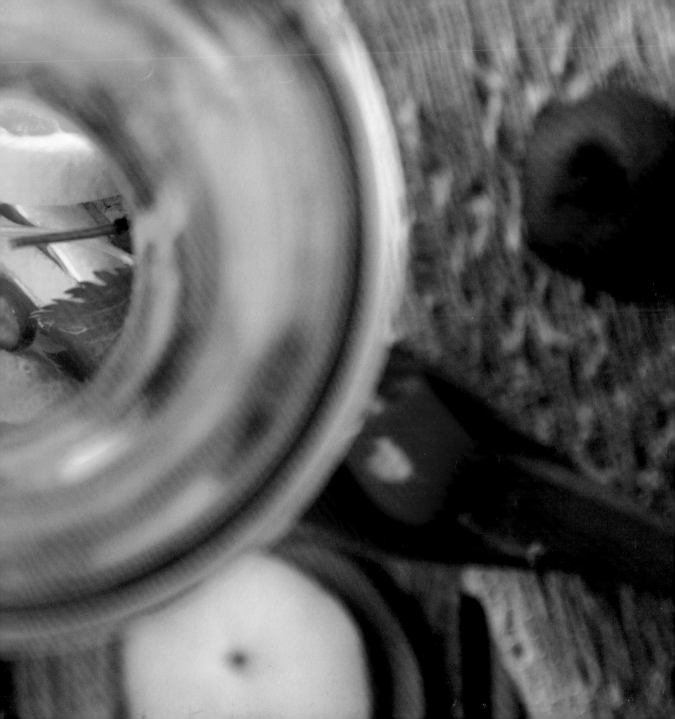

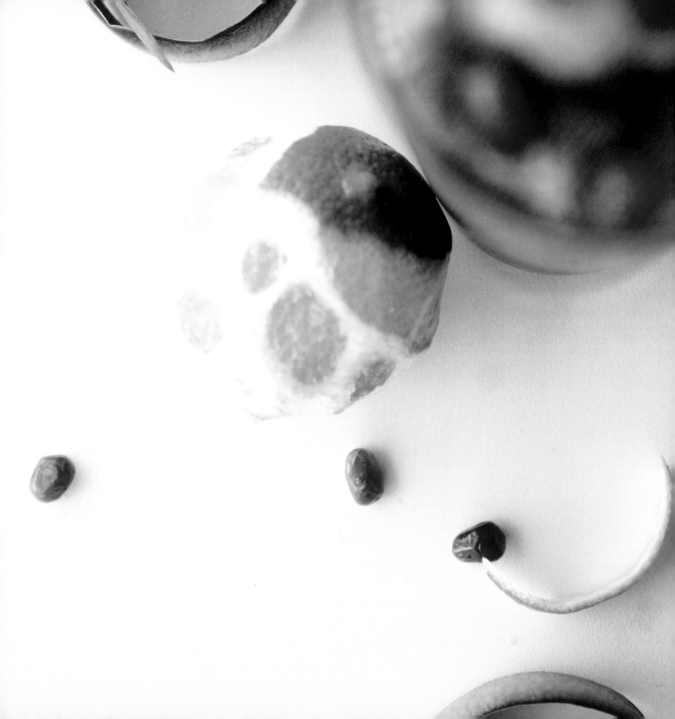

SUPERFOOD BENEFITS

M any of us have tunnel vision when it comes to seeking out health through dietary choices. We get caught up in whatever trend is sweeping the collective conversation or whatever ailment we are trying to *cure,* and we pursue singular benefits as if wholesome food is not a comprehensive nutritional package. Questions like, "What does this smoothie do for me?" are asked with the assumption, and hope, that the answer is a simple list of two or three destination-focused answers: "This one will improve your eyesight" or "This one will get rid of that acne."

Sadly, this is how a great deal of people view dietary choices with regard to health; as a series of quick, solution picking and choosing with no thought given to what else we put in our bodies on a daily basis. Perhaps this one tooth-strengthening meal will remove the effects of a lifetime caramel addiction . . . not very likely.

This is not to say that if you have a condition that requires a great deal of a specific mineral, for example, that you shouldn't seek foods that contain a higher concentration of that mineral; to do so is common sense. It is simply to say that a diet with a nutrient-dense, whole foods-focused foundation will already put you ahead of the game. I have always believed, and reality seems to concur, that a strong foundation, in all aspects of life, is better equipped to handle outliers and *dis-ease* when and if it should arise. In other words, a diet built on proper nutrition can handle a weekend of hot dogs and beer far more easily than one built on impulse and reactionary healthy eating binges.

Superfood drinks contain ingredients that provide an exceptional amount of nutrition per serving and make for a nutritional foundation with which a life full of health and wellness can flourish. While I do provide simple categorical benefits for each drink in the form of icons indicating *cleanse/detox*, *beauty*, *immune boost*, *low cal*, and *protein*, I hope my argument thus far has convinced you that each of these drinks do far more than is ascribed by its benefit icon. Some of these broader benefits include macro- and micronutrients aplenty: perfect combinations of **carbohydrates**, **fats**, and **proteins**; large amounts of **vitamins**, **minerals**, **phytochemicals**, and **enzymes**; loads of age-defying **antioxidants**; and cleansing **fiber**. All of these provide an overall increase in **energy** to boot.

We are all familiar, or at least should be, with the importance of vitamins and minerals and, at the very least, we know we should be consuming foods that are not devoid of them. They are, after all, an essential nutrient, in that our bodies cannot synthesize sufficient quantities and therefore must be obtained from the foods we eat. Since many foods in our modern, manufactured world are sorely lacking in vitamins and minerals, adding superfood drinks becomes a no-brainer.

Phytochemicals are naturally occurring chemical compounds found in plants. They are not considered essential nutrients, but research suggests they have a strong potential to impact our health nonetheless, especially where disease is concerned. Phytochemicals are mostly responsible for color and smell; the red in raspberries, the pungent smell of garlic, etc.

A general rule is the brighter a fruit or vegetable, or the more unique and pungent its smell, the more useful it is in terms of its medicinal and nutritional effects. This, of course, also works in all aspects of life; for instance, the poison dart frog has a beautiful, brightly colored body and is highly poisonous. People who often don gaudy, attention-seeking clothing and accessories generally make for an exciting event, profundity notwithstanding. People who exude generosity and kindness are said to have a sunny disposition, a heart made of gold, or a brightness to their person. It's fascinating how nature mimics itself in a variety of manifestations, but I digress. My point is that our senses *sense* extremes, and we lean toward them for a reason. Although no research has proven without a doubt that these chemicals in and of themselves are responsible for curing disease, it is well documented that eating foods high in them are essential to long-term health.

Antioxidants are more of a molecule category since they have multiple types, including vitamins, enzymes, and phytochemicals. They are generally at the forefront of all anti-aging discussions, since they inhibit the oxidation, and ultimately destruction, of cells. The short story is that oxidation creates free radicals, which in turn damage and destroy cells; antioxidants put a stop to that. Just as with phytochemicals, there is no evidence to suggest that antioxidants alone can help fight diseases like cancer, and indeed some studies show excess supplementation to be harmful in certain situations. However, it is well known and documented that foods high in antioxidants do indeed help the fight against disease—even more reasons to avoid cherry-picking foods by specific benefits and instead build a foundation of health on variety and whole foods. Superfood drinks give us those combinations in spades.

This broad array of high-quality nutrients brings with it the key to fighting almost every ailment you can imagine. Indeed, these ailments most likely stem from foods low in nutrient density, so it stands to reason that changing your diet, or at the very least introducing better choices, is the first step to eliminating disease. I would be remiss not to mention stress and exercise as the other two key components, but there is no doubt that diet is a crucial step one. The introduction of superfoods to your diet can:

- lower the risk of heart disease
- help with eczema and psoriasis
- regulate blood pressure
- balance cholesterol
- reduce bad bacterial growth
- reduce or eliminate cancer cell growth
- reduce viral growth
- eliminate headaches
- help with insomnia
- reduce or eliminate bowel issues

Energy is another big bonus to consuming superfood drinks. They are brimming with nutrients and, if you add fruit (sugar), you can expect an eye-opening boost of energy akin to caffeine—*without* the jitters. This is the most palpable benefit of superfood drinks and, naturally, the one that informs folks they are actually working. The effect on your psyche should be apparent as well; since you know you are doing good by your body, your mind will reward you with a feeling of accomplishment that will manifest through your physical being in the form of clarity and increased energy. After all, the mind *is* the body.

Superfood drinks can also be the missing link to weight management, whether your goal is to increase or decrease. I will go into this topic further in the chapter titled *Diets,* but suffice to say that adding a superfood drink packed with protein can be a welcome addition to your post-workout routine for repairing and building muscle as well as a way to curb hunger and replace bad food choices when that hunger manifests. Feeding your body what it actually needs is a great way to eliminate or suppress cravings that cause overeating and ultimately unwanted weight gain.

A huge bonus for me was what it did for my indigestion woes. For many years, I suffered from mild heartburn and acid indigestion, and the thought of medication seemed to me a lazy way to avoid the problem with a pseudo-solution. Within weeks of adding superfood drinks—green smoothies, to be specific— my indigestion was nearly non-existent. Keeping with the routine of highly alkalizing greens and the elimination of trigger foods in the rest of my diet, the problem went away entirely. Now, I can safely have the occasional pasta with red sauce, and my body is able to cope without fists full of antacids.

With superfood drinks, it is quick and easy to combine high-quality macronutrients—carbs, fats, and protein—into a complete, on-the-go meal. Our superfood ingredients are chosen specifically because they contain a larger amount of micronutrients—vitamins, minerals, phytochemicals, antioxidants—than most foods typically do. These ingredients really pack a punch.

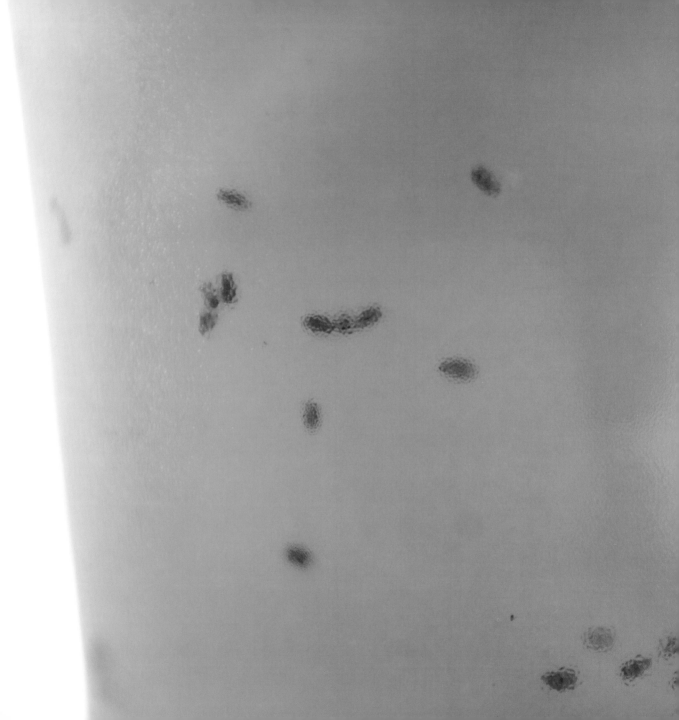

SMOOTHIES VERSUS JUICES

First, let us remember that we are essentially discussing the merits of two incredibly beneficial and healthy ways of consuming vital nutrients. There are no losers here when either choice is a definite win for your body and mind. When in doubt, have a smoothie—it's quicker, cheaper, and more satiating. Now, let us discover *the lesser of two goods*, if you will.

OXIDATION

This is the meeting of a substance, in this case our superfood drink ingredients, with oxygen. Why is oxidation an important factor to consider?

Food begins to decompose the second it meets oxygen; one can conclude, then, that all food, and indeed all life, is in a slow state of decomposition the moment it has reached its pinnacle. With regard to fruits and vegetables, that high point is what we call *ripe*.

The protective layer, i.e. the skin, helps to slow this decomposition down. However, as soon as they are opened, whether by knife, blender blade, or juicer gears, the decomposition is dramatically increased. This is why avocados, for example, turn brown shortly after being cut. Decomposition means the cells are beginning to die. Dead cells mean fewer nutrients, and fewer nutrients mean a whole lot of nothing in terms of giving your body what it needs to thrive.

Making a smoothie requires one to add ingredients to a blender that then breaks open these ingredients, causing oxidation to increase for the very reasons mentioned previously. Oxidation is further increased by the very nature of blender mechanics; it whips air (oxygen) into the smoothie. However, we must also consider that smoothies do not eliminate the fibrous material like juicing does. This fibrous material, with its cell walls broken open, allows more antioxidants to release into the drink and decreases the rate at which the smoothie oxidizes, hence *anti*-oxidant.

Juicing oxidizes faster than blending. The separation, and ultimately elimination, of fibrous material leaves you with essentially water, vitamins, enzymes, and minerals that are susceptible to oxidation in greater effect. Furthermore, the type of juicer you use can play a role. A centrifugal juicer (the most common on the market) does not extract the most optimal amount of juice, and therefore does not break open cell walls nearly as well for that precious antioxidant boost. Triturating juicers, however, are the most expensive juicers on the market, have a much slower movement, and extract every drop of juice available while causing overall nutrients to increase. Those familiar with using the different types of juicers will notice centrifugal-made juice is best consumed right away, and triturating-made juice can last almost twice as long.

Unconvinced? Try a simple experiment: blend an apple in one cup and juice an apple in another. Which one changes color (browns) first? The juice. For my money, I'd rather get the whole deal—fiber and all—with a delicious smoothie, but to each her own.

NUTRITIONAL BOOST

The difference here is speed and quantity. Because juicing eliminates all fibrous material and because one must juice two to three times as many ingredients to achieve a similar quantity, we are left with a highly concentrated elixir of vitamins, minerals, and enzymes that enter the bloodstream significantly faster and to greater effect. This is why I have always believed it is important to limit your juice serving sizes much smaller than those for smoothies.

ENERGY BOOST

As with the nutritional boost, we have a significantly higher amount of sugar concentrated in juices than we do with smoothies. The energy boost you get is somewhat related to the increase in nutrients, but the brunt of that charge is led by sugar, plain and simple. And if experience has taught us anything, we know that with a great, energizing sugar rush comes a great midday nap.

COST EFFECTIVENESS

Expect to spend upward of three to four times the amount of money keeping a strict juicing regimen than you would for smoothies. One apple goes a long way in the blender, but in the juicer, it's a few sips. It's even worse for green, leafy vegetables, unless you're lucky enough to have a triturating juicer. Even then, you'd be hard pressed to get a cup of juice from an entire bag of fresh, organic greens. I use juicing more as a treat, or when I want to add a bit of something to my smoothies that won't take well to a blender: carrots, beets, etc.

SENSITIVE STOMACHS

Digestion issues are no fun, but that doesn't mean we have to sacrifice easy nutrition because of it. This is the only category in which the preference is pointed toward juices rather than smoothies. The fiber in smoothies can cause irritation of the stomach lining, depending on your condition and the fruits and vegetables used, so it is important to slowly introduce new combinations to see what works and what doesn't. Juices are easier on the digestive system, but it is still important to use caution, as some combinations of starchy vegetables can cause excess gas in some people. Every body is different, so start slow and see what you can handle.

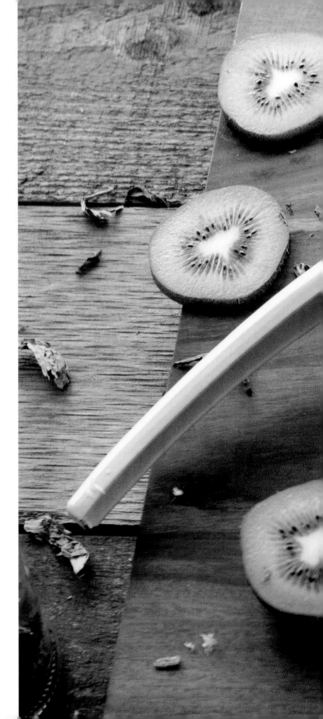

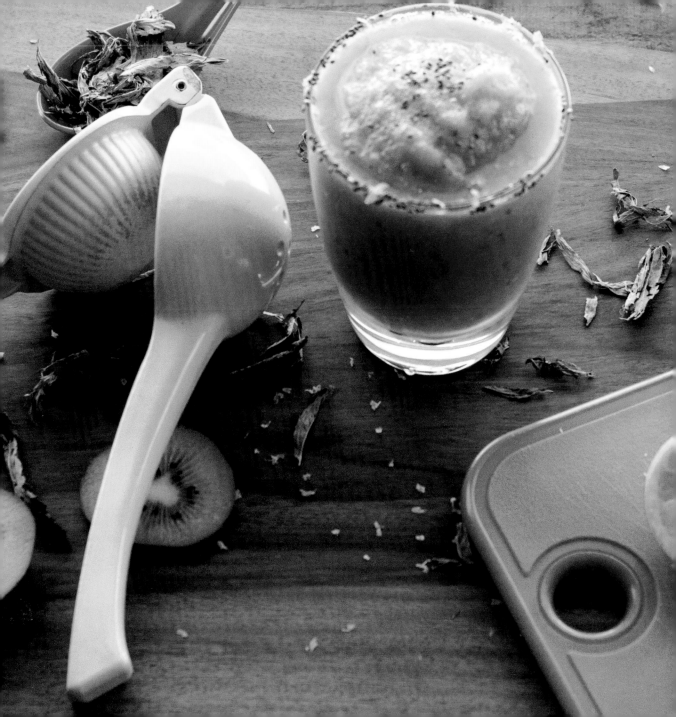

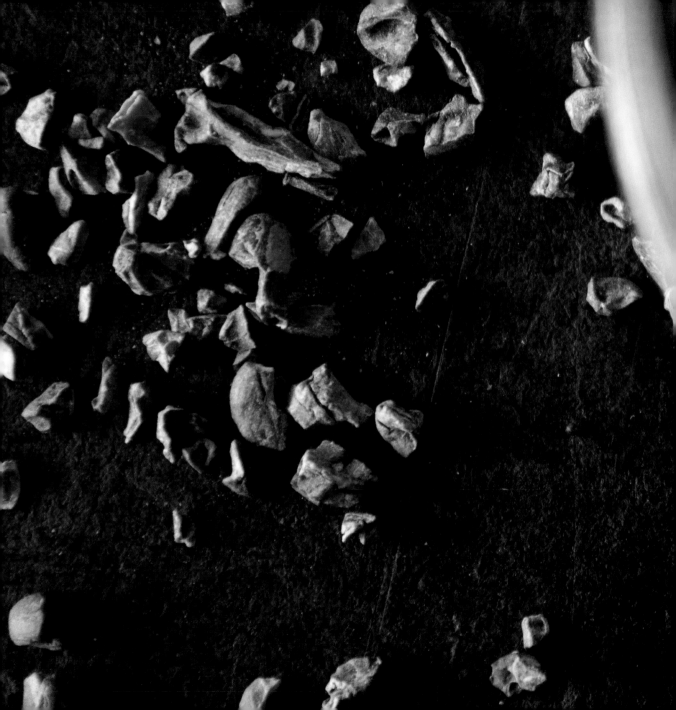

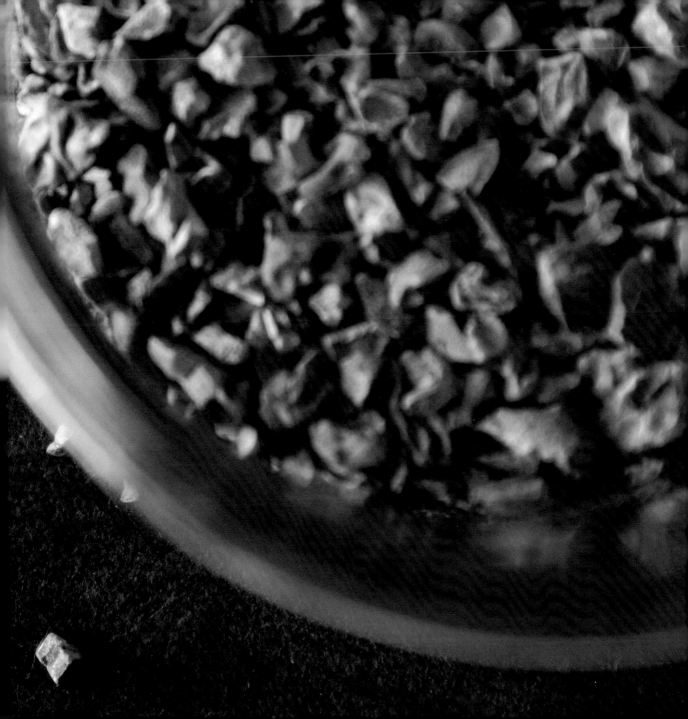

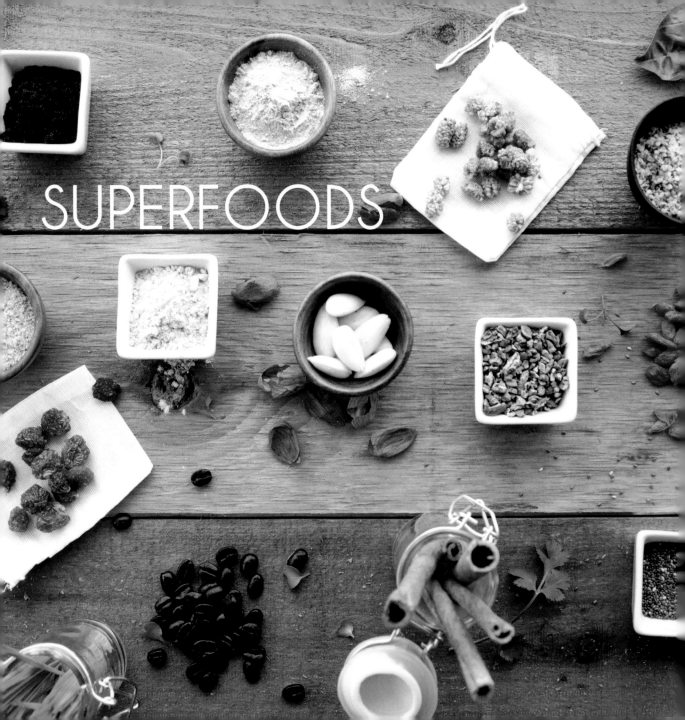

SUPERFOODS

SUPERFOOD INGREDIENTS

Hate to break it to you, but the actual word *superfood* is simply a marketing term used to describe foods that are beneficial to your health. There is nothing special about them outside of that very broad definition. An apple, for example, is technically a superfood. Some definitions reach even further by claiming they may help certain medical conditions, but as I alluded to in the benefits chapter, we know that no one food is responsible for healing specific ailments. It is a balanced diet with a foundation of nutrient-dense foods that halts disease and allows us to thrive—a foundation consisting of a variety of superfoods.

Despite the term being used for marketing, we cannot deny the effect it has had on the health food market, nor can we deny the need for singling out healthy foods from manufactured, low-quality food. The following are simply superfoods that lend themselves particularly well to drinks like smoothies, juices, coffees, and teas.

SUPERHEROES

These are ingredients typically found on superfood lists; some are exotic, perhaps, but all are relatively affordable and available in most health food stores, and certainly online. You don't need *all* of these, but I encourage you to experiment with perhaps a few per month to introduce new flavors and keep your diet as varied as possible.

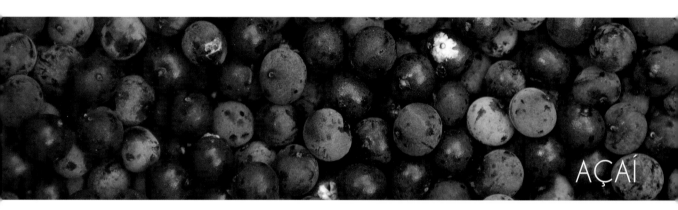

AÇAÍ

Serving Size: 1 tbsp. powder

I suppose we can thank Oprah for the upsurge of açaí popularity here in the United States, but despite the claims you often hear for this *magical fruit*, it is not exceptionally different than other berries you have no doubt come across, like blueberries, which are also on this superfoods list. It does, however, contain slightly higher amounts of antioxidants than typical North American berries and is also considered a *fatty fruit*, in that it contains a good amount of healthy fats. For those reasons, it deserves a place of its own. Açaí is a common fruit in Brazil and other parts of South America and can be enjoyed in its natural, fresh-from-the-tree form, as opposed to the frozen purées and powders we get in the United States. It is a small, round, black-purple fruit that grows from the tall, slender açaí palm native to Central and South America. It has a rich blackberry and dark chocolate flavor and a somewhat grainy texture and pairs well with coconut, milk, bananas, and nuts. It's pronounced *ah-sigh-ee*.

Benefits: Açaí is a low-sugar fruit with high levels of antioxidants. It may promote longevity and is great for those wishing to keep their sugar consumption low. It also contains a number of healthy fats and has a rich vitamin and mineral content.

Where to Buy: Unfortunately, açaí does not travel well in its berry form so, in the United States, we rarely have access to them in that way. Instead, look for purées in the frozen food section of your local health food store and make sure they contain no added sugar. This is the best option, since the flavor is retained quite well. The next best option, which we use throughout this book, is the freeze-dried powder form. This should also be sugar-free and usually contains vitamin C (citric acid) to preserve the fats. Both forms should be organic. If you happen to visit Brazil, try the delicious, smoothie-like *açaí na tigela*, found in stands along the coastline.

SEAWEEDS

Algae (spirulina & chlorella)
Serving Size: 1 tsp. powder

The two most popular forms of what is known as *blue-green algae* are spirulina and chlorella. To note, they are technically not algaes, but cyanobacteria, a form of bacteria that obtain their energy through photosynthesis.

Both are both powerful cleansing supplements and have very strong and distinct flavor profiles. For this reason, it is best to start with lower servings to test your tolerance. It is also best to limit consumption to a few times per month at most to detoxify the body as needed. Citrus and other strong flavors work well when adding algae to superfood drinks.

Benefits: Spirulina and especially chlorella are one of the most nutritionally concentrated foods we can consume. They both are made of more than 50 percent protein with a complete amino acid profile and are high in fatty acids such as omega-3 DHA and EPA. They are widely known for having excellent detox properties, as they bind to heavy metals and other toxins to assist in their elimination. They contain a wide variety of vitamins and minerals and are considered to be one of the best supplements for boosting the immune system, improving digestion, and normalizing blood pressure.

Where to Buy: Spirulina and chlorella can be found in most health food stores or online. Be sure to look for organic versions, along with other purity designators. The cell walls of chlorella are indigestible, so it is important to find varieties that refer to "broken-cell wall" or "cracked wall," so the nutrients inside are bioavailable.

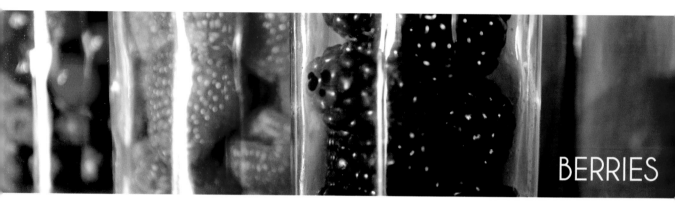

BERRIES

Serving Size: 1 cup

Blueberries, blackberries, raspberries, strawberries, and cranberries are some of the more common North American berries with which you are no doubt familiar. There are, in fact, thousands of different strains, though, and I encourage you to seek out unfamiliar varieties such as currants, gooseberries, elderberries, and lingonberries. Berries have a wide variety of flavor profiles and work in just about any smoothie, juice, or infused water.

Benefits: As evidenced by their often bright and colorful skins, berries contain a wide variety of pigments that have been known to be potent antioxidants. They are also high in many vitamins, including the immune boosters C and A.

Where to Buy: Organic berries can be found at local farmers' markets, health food stores, supermarkets, and even sidewalk fruit stands. Since berries, along with greens, are typically blasted with a high amount of pesticides, it is important to always buy organic. During the summer season, they can be purchased fresh at a reduced cost, but otherwise it is most cost-effective to buy frozen. I have saved hundreds of dollars throughout the years thanks to Trader Joe's organic frozen blueberries.

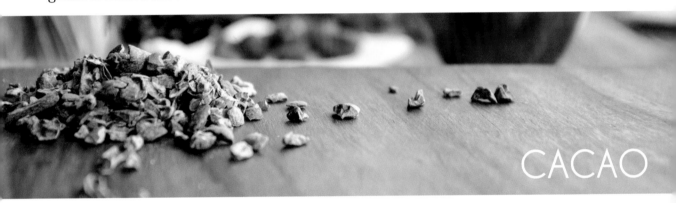

CACAO

Serving Size: 2 tbsp. nibs or powder

Raw chocolate, need I say more? Okay, I'll say a bit more. Chocolate is not only a powerful nutrient source, but also well-loved and known as a dessert food. In this way, we can use its raw form, cacao, to mimic less nutritious sugar-filled drinks. It works great with milks, bananas, avocados, berries, oranges, vanilla bean, and cinnamon. There are two forms of cacao that work well in superfood smoothies. My favorite is cacao nibs, which are broken pieces of the whole cacao bean. They do not blend completely and lend a fantastic, crunchy texture to the drink. The other form is cacao powder, which blends well and has a stronger flavor.

Do not confuse raw cacao with cocoa. Although they are very similar, the latter is usually roasted and contains less of a nutrient punch. Avoid all varieties with added sugar.

Benefits: Cacao is an extremely rich source of antioxidants (more than most berries) as well as flavonoids, which have been shown to benefit cardiovascular health as well as brain function. It's also rich in minerals like magnesium (great for post-workout) and calcium. It is also a stimulant, due to a compound called theobromine, which has been shown to support emotional and mental health.

Where to Buy: Cacao powder and cacao nibs can be found online or at most health food stores. Be sure to buy unroasted, sugar-free, preferably organic, and fair-trade varieties.

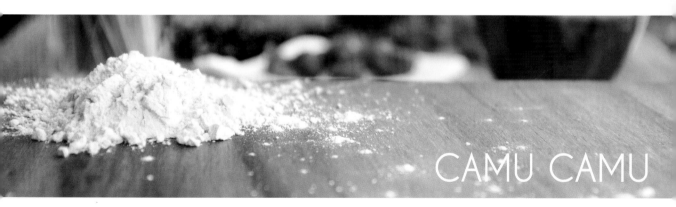

CAMU CAMU

Serving Size: 1 tsp. powder

Camu berries, commonly referred to as camu camu, are native to Peru and Brazil. They are extremely acidic in berry form and best used in smoothies with the addition of other sweet fruits to balance the tartness. They can be added to almost any superfood drink to give it a significant vitamin C boost. These work well with herbs and stevia.

Benefits: These berries are extremely high in vitamin C; in fact they have the second highest vitamin C concentration of any fruit, almost twenty times that of an orange. This makes them a perfect superfood for those wanting to boost their immune system to fight off colds.

Where to Buy: In the United States, we are unfortunately unable to get fresh camu camu berries, so we must purchase organic powder from health food stores or online outlets.

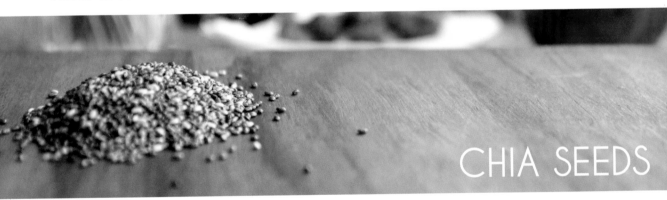

CHIA SEEDS

Serving Size: 2 tbsp. seeds

These are one of my favorite superfoods—and not only because they are reminiscent of tiny dinosaur eggs. They are very small seeds that come from a plant in the mint family native to southern Mexico and Guatemala. The seeds are mucilaginous so, when soaked in liquid, they retain the liquid, creating an almost jelly-like texture that suspends itself in whatever drink you add it to. They can be added to superfood drinks as a thickening agent by either adding the seeds and letting the mixture sit for twenty minutes, or by pre-soaking the seeds in water to form a gel that can be spooned in to your desired consistency.

Benefits: Rich in omega-3 fatty acids, chia seeds have long been used to boost energy. They are high in fiber, protein, minerals, and antioxidants. They are a low-calorie food that supports healthy digestion. Adding them to coconut water creates a perfect post-run refreshment.

Where to Buy: Chia seeds are found online or at your local health food markets. There are two types: seeds and powders. The recipes in this book use the seeds, as I find them to have a pleasant texture.

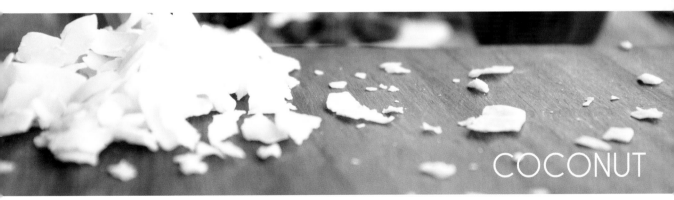

COCONUT

Serving Size: 1 cup water; 2 tbsp. oil

Coconut is one of nature's miracle foods, and with good reason: the benefits are wide and diverse. From the simple coconut, we get many ingredient variations that lend themselves to superfood drinks quite well: oil, creamy milk, and sweet water, as well as the meat, which can provide delicious chewy bits in smoothies. When adding oil to drinks, it's best to melt it first to avoid clumping. Coconut water can be substituted for water in almost any superfood drink to add an electrolyte boost.

Benefits: Coconut has been used for everything from skin care to treating heart disease; lowering blood pressure and cholesterol levels; for weight loss by increasing metabolism; for those with digestive issues; and even as a primary ingredient in infant formulas. Coconut water is great for post-workout to replenish electrolytes, and coconut oil makes a wonderful cooking oil with a high smoke point.

Where to Buy: Most markets sell some form of coconut: organic virgin coconut oil, whole young coconuts, organic pure coconut milk, or pure coconut water.

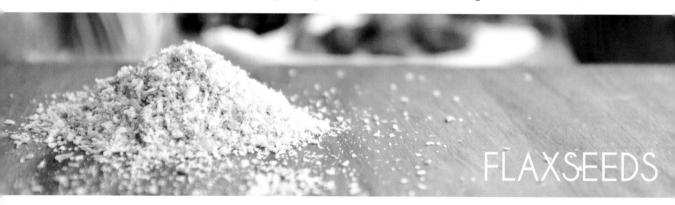

FLAXSEEDS

Serving Size: 2 tbsp. ground powder

Flaxseed is probably the most popular and well-known superfood in this bunch. It has a very mild, nutty flavor that is masked by most other ingredients. It must be eaten in its ground form, otherwise the seed will pass through undigested. Add it to any smoothie for a boost of fatty acids.

Benefits: Flaxseed is a great source of fiber. It contains short-chain omega-3 fatty acids called alpha-linolenic acid (ALA), which is both a powerful antioxidant and has been known to reduce anxiety and stress. It is also rich in lignans, which have been known to reduce the risk of breast and prostate cancer, and high in vitamin E, making it a great choice for the skin health.

Where to Buy: Flaxseed comes in the whole seed form or pre-ground powders. It is much more cost effective to buy the whole seeds and use a coffee grinder to make your own powder. Flaxseed oil can oxidize and go rancid quickly, so store your powders in the refrigerator or freezer. Find them at your local health food stores.

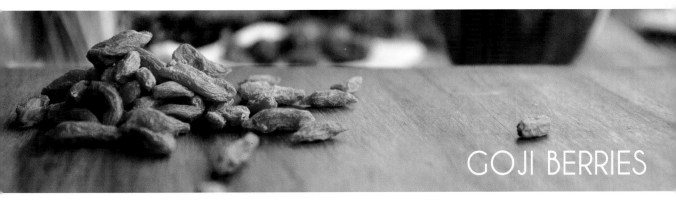

GOJI BERRIES

Serving Size: 2–3 tbsp. dried berries

Goji berries, also known as wolfberries, are native to southeastern Europe and

Asia. They are a bright orange-red and most often found in dried form in the United States. They have a slightly sweet and sour flavor and plump nicely when soaked for ten minutes. They blend well with almost anything.

Benefits: Commonly used to treat high blood pressure and diabetes in Chinese medicine, they are great sources of vitamin C and E and have been used to boost energy levels and support healthy vision, as well as increase metabolism.

Where to Buy: Dried goji berries can be found at most health food stores or online. Be sure to buy organic. Freshly dried goji berries are bright in color and have a chewy texture. Avoid varieties with added sugar.

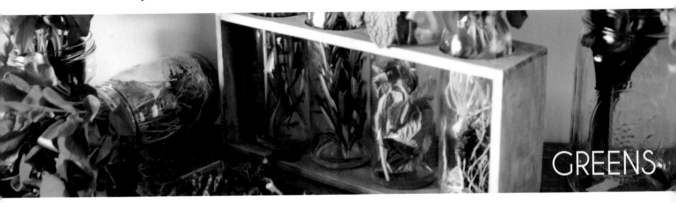

GREENS

Serving Size: 2 cups, packed

We're talking just about any green, leafy vegetable you can think of: spinach, kale, chard, lettuce, watercress, oregano, basil, mint, cilantro, broccoli, wheat-grass, and many more. Because they are so low in calories, you'll find it difficult to eat too much.

Superfood drinks are my preferred way of getting my daily vegetable requirement and, as a bonus, the other ingredients in the drinks often mask or change flavors I don't usually prefer, thereby increasing the variety and nutrition I receive.

Benefits: Greens are some of the most nutritionally dense foods on the planet while remaining significantly low in calories. High in cancer-fighting antioxidants, vitamins, minerals, fiber, and even protein, they are also alkaline foods and can help with ailments like indigestion, eczema and psoriasis, and bad bacterial growth.

Where to Buy: Greens can be grown, purchased from local farmers' markets, or found at almost any grocery store. Always seek out organic greens to maximize nutrients and minimize potentially harmful pesticides.

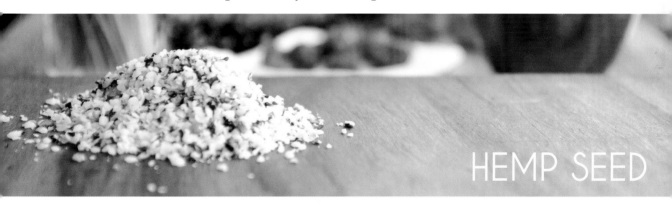

HEMP SEED

Serving Size: 2–3 tbsp. hulled seeds

Edible hemp seeds (without THC) are not to be confused with marijuana seeds (with THC). They are small seeds that can be eaten raw, made into milk, or ground into a powder. The taste is nutty and very similar to a blend of pine nuts and sunflower seeds. Any post-workout smoothie will benefit from adding hemp seeds or powder.

Benefits: Hemp seeds are one of the best sources of plant protein around, which is why the ground form is often labeled as *hemp protein powder* rather than just hemp powder. It contains all known amino acids (including the essential 9), about 80 percent essential fatty acids (including omega-3, omega-6, and GLA), and a wide variety of beneficial vitamins and minerals.

Where to Buy: Look for raw, hulled seed varieties or powders (often labeled as hemp protein powder) with no additives at your local health food store. Organic is a plus, but not necessary, as hemp crops typically use very little to no pesticides.

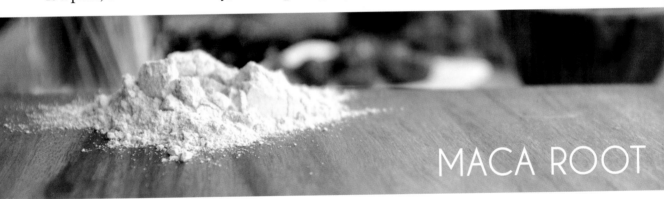

MACA ROOT

Serving Size: 1 tbsp. powder

Maca is a root native to the high Andes of Peru, where it thrives in one of the highest farming regions in the world. Because of its hearty nature, it retains most of its nutrients long after being refined into a powder for consumption. It has a potent nutty, bitter, and radish-like flavor that may take some getting used to. It works well with milks, bananas, dried mulberries, and almonds.

Benefits: Maca root has been used for thousands of years as a potent aphrodisiac, doubling libidio in some recent clinical trials. It is also known to balance hormone levels, thereby reducing stress and increasing energy. It's also loaded with amino acids, vitamins, minerals, protein, and fiber.

Where to Buy: Look for the raw, whole root powder in local health food stores or online.

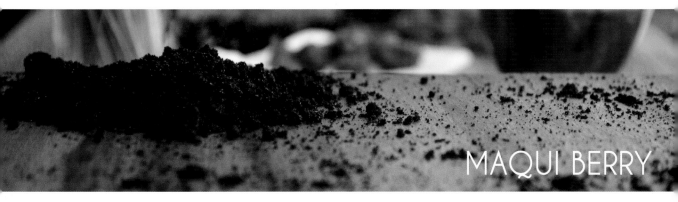

MAQUI BERRY

Serving Size: 2 tsp. powder

Maqui berries are similar in size and appearance to blueberries and have a slightly muted blackberry flavor. They are native to the rainforests of Chile and southern Argentina. The powder, which we use in the recipes in this book, is a very vivid purple and, because the flavor is so mild, it goes well with almost anything.

Benefits: Traditionally, maqui has been used to treat diarrhea, fever, or inflammation. It was used by the Mapuche Indians to boost strength and stamina. It has one of the highest antioxidant levels of any fruit and contains high levels of vitamin C.

Where to Buy: In the United States, we only have access to dried maqui berry powder. Look for freeze-dried varieties at your local health food store or online. Maqui is another ingredient that should be stored in a sealed container in the refrigerator or freezer because it oxidizes quickly.

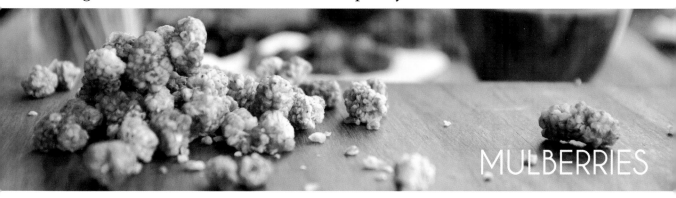

MULBERRIES

Serving Size: 2–3 tbsp. dried berries

Mulberries look like elongated raspberries or blackberries. The white mulberry is an east Asian species that has all but taken over in North America. It has a milder flavor than the dark varieties and, when dried (as we use in the recipes in this book), it takes on a very sweet vanilla-like flavor. It also works well as a granola substitute on yogurt.

Benefits: The stem bark of the mulberry plant has a significant amount of resveratrol, which translates to the fruit, although not as potent. Resveratrol is said to have powerful anti-aging properties. They contain half the sugar in most dried fruits yet still lend a sweet flavor. They are a great source of protein and are high in colon-cleansing fiber.

Where to Buy: Find sun-dried white mulberries at your local health food stores. Fresh mulberries may be available but are less desirable when adding to smoothies. The dried varieties are sweet and chewy.

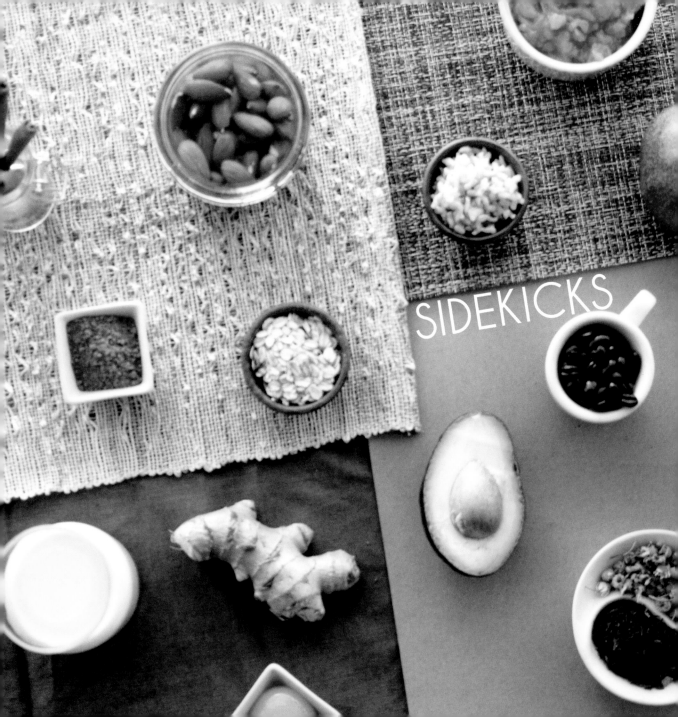

SIDEKICKS

SIDEKICKS

Some of these ingredients don't always make the typical superfoods list, but certainly should, and others you'll recognize as being a *must-eat food*. Combining them with one another, or especially with ingredients on the *superheroes* list, can make for a complete meal in terms of macro- and micronutrient density, along with increasing flavor and providing a more appealing texture.

Superheroes are essential to superfood drinks, and *sidekicks* are recommended, but together they are the ideal choice.

The Combo

The *combo* is what I call two or more sidekicks. Adding two or more lesser known healthy foods or ingredients that are not as nutrient-dense as foods typically referred to as superfoods makes for a superfood itself in my book. Green tea with ginger? Superfood. Grass-fed butter and coffee? Superfood. You get the idea.

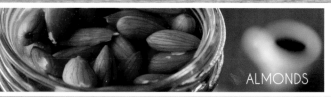

ALMONDS

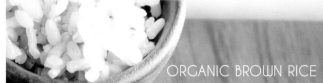

ORGANIC BROWN RICE

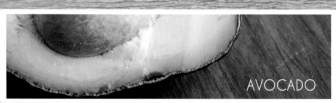

AVOCADO

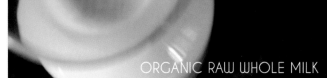

ORGANIC RAW WHOLE MILK

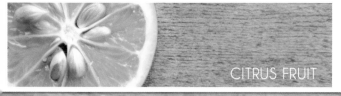

CINNAMON

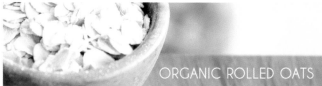

ORGANIC ROLLED OATS

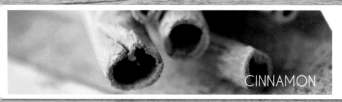

CITRUS FRUIT

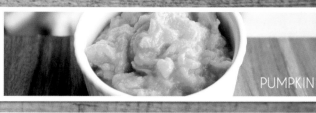

PUMPKIN

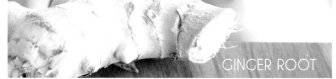

GINGER ROOT

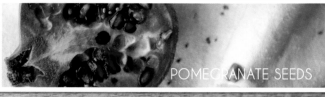

POMEGRANATE SEEDS

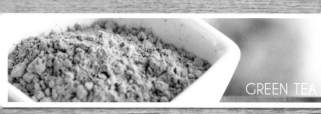

GREEN TEA

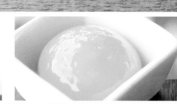

PASTURED EGG YOLKS

Avocado: One of the healthiest sources of monounsaturated fats, it helps absorption of vitamins, minerals, and antioxidants in the other ingredients used in your drink. It also provides a creamy texture to your superfood drinks.

Cinnamon: It has an antimicrobial effect that eliminates bad breath and impairs tumor growth, and it's great for colon health. It also has a flavor profile that lends itself to almost anything. Look for Ceylon or Saigon varieties.

Citrus Fruits: Packed with vitamin C, these are great for boosting the immune system.

Coffee Beans: Caffeine is known to boost concentration, enhance memory, and increase energy. These are great for pre-workout, and they have also shown to curb Alzheimer's, dementia, and Parkinson's.

Ginger Root: This ingredient is great for nausea (especially during pregnancy) and gastric illnesses. It also helps to ease muscle pain and eliminate inflammation. One of the best remedies for symptoms of the cold and flu is ginger combined with oregano oil. Use fresh ginger root and juice or freeze the root and shave it right into the drink with a zester.

Grass-Fed Butter: Always use grass-fed (and preferably organic) butter. Butter made from grain-fed cows is inferior in many ways: it does not blend well, the fat content is weighted towards the unhealthy side, and flavor suffers. Grass-fed butter has a higher vitamin content, a better fatty acid composition (omega-3 and -6 are equal), and a higher conjugated linoleic acid (CLA) content that has been linked to heart health and fat loss. *Kerrygold* is a great, widely available brand.

Green Tea: This ingredient has been linked to a great deal of health benefits including fighting cancer and arthritis, boosting immunity, and better overall cardiovascular health. The recipes in this book use organic matcha green tea powder; a little goes a long way.

Organic Brown Rice: This complex carbohydrate is packed with fiber and is nutrient-dense. It's also filling while remaining low in calories.

Organic Pasture-Raised Eggs: These eggs come from hens that feed on organic, non-GMO food and have access to open fields where they can graze on plants and insects aplenty. This increases the nutrition in each egg tremendously. Do not confuse this with free range or vegetarian fed.

Organic Pumpkin: Packed with carotenoids that may help fight free-radicals, these pumpkins are great for keeping the skin looking and feeling young. They contain more potassium than a banana. Look for organic canned 100 percent pure pumpkin purée.

Organic Rolled Oats: This is another complex carbohydrate with high protein levels and fiber. It's a nutrient-dense food that supports healthy digestion.

Organic Whole Milk Yogurt: Same great nutritional benefits as milk, but with the added bonus of healthy gut bacteria in the form of probiotics. Lactose intolerant people often find they can consume yogurt without issue, since the lactose in yogurt is partially converted to glucose and galactose.

Organic Raw Milk: Raw milk has a higher nutritional content and better flavor. Most people previously diagnosed with lactose intolerance no longer suffer symptoms when switching to raw, and purchasing this milk means you'll be supporting local farmers. The risk of developing serious illness because the milk hasn't been pasteurized is ridiculously small: about 1 in 6 million. In fact, according to recent studies, you are four times more likely to become ill from produce than you are from raw milk.

Pomegranate Seeds: High in vitamin C and K and rich in anti-cancer, heart-healthy phytochemicals that have been shown to lower blood pressure and reduce inflammation.

Raw Almonds: These are a good source of protein, manganese, potassium, copper, vitamin E, and monounsaturated fats. Studies also suggest that almonds can reduce the risk of gallstones.

Turmeric: A great anti-inflammatory, turmeric has been shown to help with arthritis and prevent Alzheimer's. It is also an effective cancer fighter and can reduce muscle soreness after a workout.

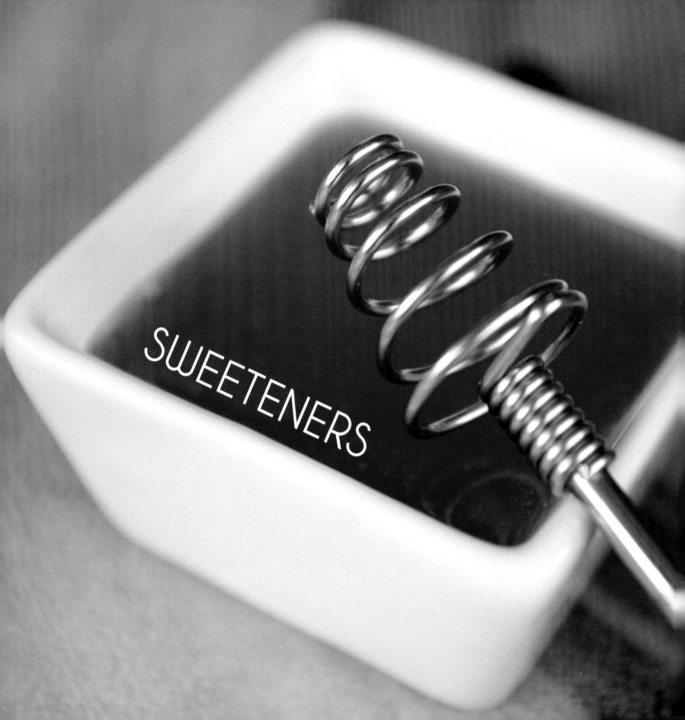

SWEETENERS

Throughout the recipes in this book, and as a general rule in your overall diet, I recommend using only natural sources of unprocessed sweeteners. The primary source should come from fruit; bananas, dates, figs, apples, pears, peaches, and nectarines are some of the more common fruits that can add varying degrees of sweetness to your drinks. If the particular recipe does not accommodate these fruits, or if your sweet tooth is particularly insistent, the following will fit the bill.

Honey: Along with providing an almost instant energy boost, honey contains vitamins, minerals, pollen, and protein—something you won't find in granulated white sugar. The pollen has even been known to minimize seasonal allergies. Look for unfiltered, raw varieties at your local farmers' market. The sweetness factor goes a long way with honey, so a teaspoon or two should be sufficient.

Stevia: This is the most recent sugar substitute everyone is crazy about, and for good reason. Stevia or sweetleaf is a flowering plant mostly grown for its sweet leaves, which are used dried or made into extracts and powders as a natural sugar substitute. It's a great sweetener for diabetics and has even been used in the treatment of type-2 diabetics in parts of Asia. It has also been known to normalize blood pressure. It can be found in a dried leaf variety in many tea shops and health food stores. If that is unavailable, look for the *pure* powder form or liquid extract. Trader Joe's has a great organic liquid stevia extract and a 100 percent pure powder extract.

AVOID THESE!

Commercial big-name smoothie and juice establishments, as well as pre-packaged or bottled supermarket drinks, often use ingredients that completely defeat the purpose of consuming a *healthy* liquid meal.

Buying organic and fresh is best when it comes to getting the most nutrition for your money, so let's not sabotage your wholesome goals; skip the following ingredients, as the negatives outweigh any positives:

- Artificial colors and flavors
- Artificial sweeteners
- Cane sugar or cane juice
- Corn syrup or corn sugar
- Raw eggs that are **not** pastured or pasture-raised
- Soy milk and protein powders
- Juices that are bottled and pasteurized

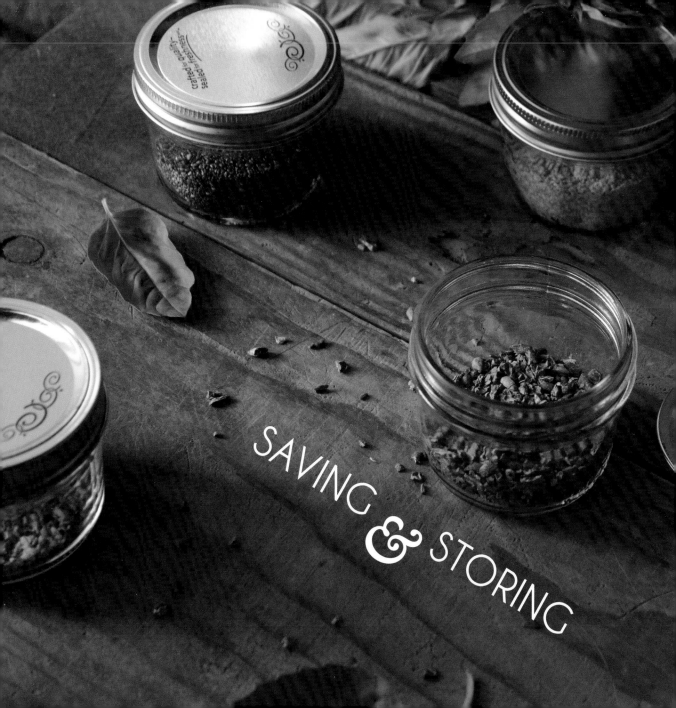

SAVING & STORING

SAVING & STORING

The most cost-effective option for fruits and vegetables is probably growing your own. However, considering that time is money, and depending on the cost of watering and feeding your plants, not to mention your location and access to space, it may or may not be cheaper for you to go this route. Sprouting seeds for herbs is an exception, as this can be done cheaply and in minimal space wherever you are.

Your next best option is buying berries and even some vegetables frozen and in bulk. Ingredients are less expensive this way, and often even fresher than their non-frozen counterparts (frozen ingredients are typically harvested, frozen, packaged, and shipped much more quickly than it takes fresh ingredients to arrive at the market).

Other great ways to save on ingredients: buy directly from local farmers and farmers' markets, and buy only fruits and vegetables that are in season.

Storing your superfoods differs depending on the ingredient, but the following points should cover all you need to know:

- Never pre-wash your fruits or vegetables, as they mold and wilt much more quickly.
- Keep most fruits on the countertop. Ripe avocados can be refrigerated to slow the decaying process.

- Store (unwashed) greens in plastic bags in the refrigerator. Some herbs like basil should not be stored in the refrigerator (herbs are easy to grow, so they should be grown fresh in a windowsill anyway).
- If a fruit or vegetable can't be eaten before going bad, cut it up, put it into a sealed plastic bag (removing as much air as possible), and toss it into the freezer.
- Powders and dried fruit are best stored in sealed mason jars in a dark, dry cupboard.
- Nuts, seeds, and dried fatty fruits like açaí are best stored in sealed mason jars in either the refrigerator or freezer.

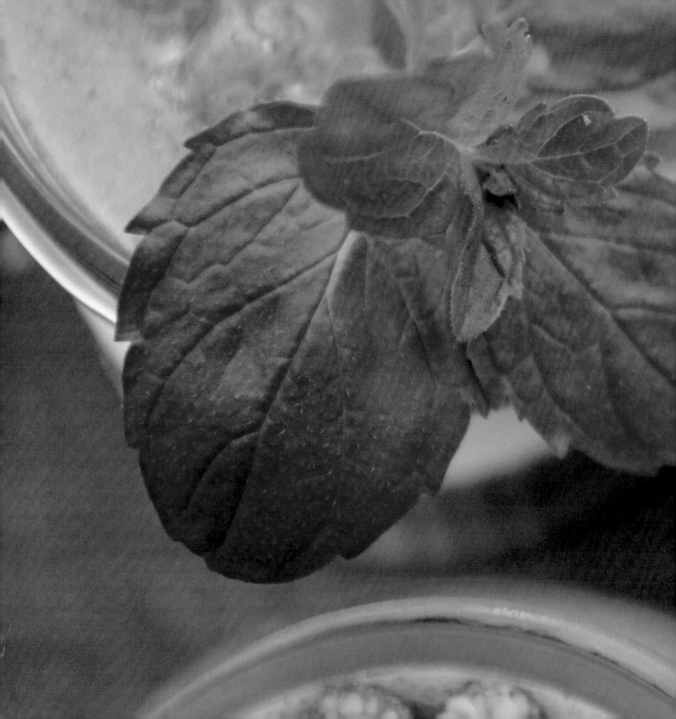

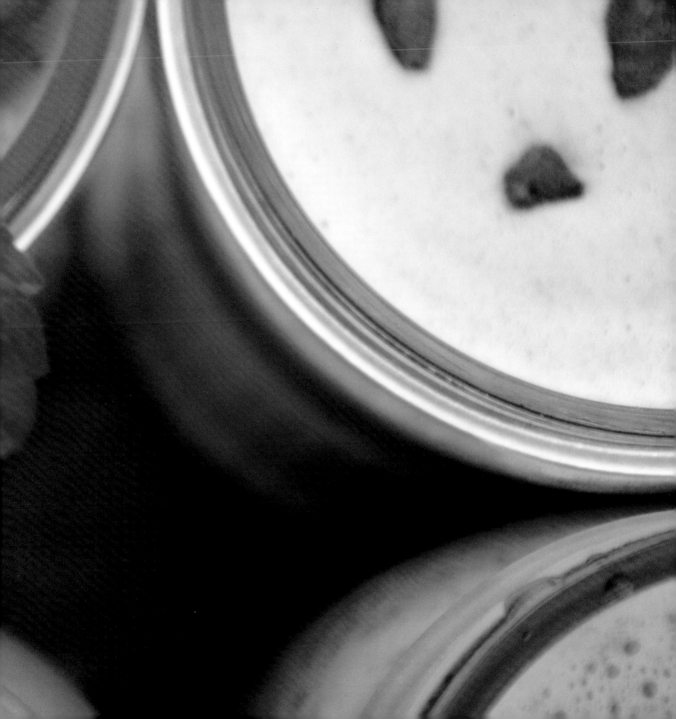

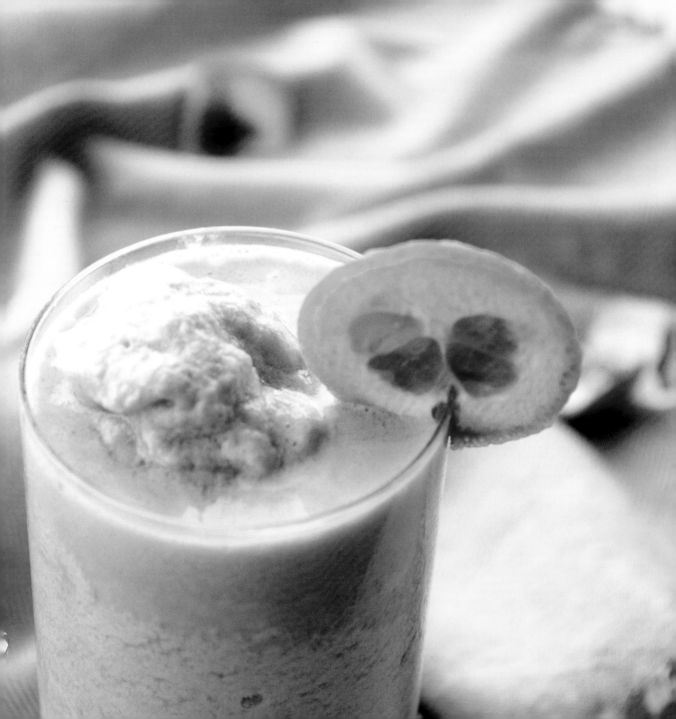

SUPERFOOD DRINK BASICS

To make use of *all* the recipes in this book, you are required to have access to both a blender and a juicer. A blender is typically a more commonplace kitchen appliance, as well as more affordable than a juicer. Because of this, and the reasons listed in the Smoothies Versus Juices chapter, I have included more smoothie recipes than juice recipes. Furthermore, most of the juice recipes also make use of a blender (to incorporate superfood powders and blend in ice). So if you own a juicer but not a blender, well, it may be time to purchase that blender. If you own a blender but not a juicer, it's up to you whether to spring for one; you'll get enough out of this book without it, to be sure. Bottom line, **a blender is a must.** I'll go over my blender recommendations in the following section.

Optional: There are coffee and tea recipes as well, so something to steep with is useful. A good chef's knife and cutting board are key elements in an efficiently (even minimally) outfitted kitchen, so you should already have these. Ice cube trays for making *super-flavored* ice, a citrus zester, mason jars for storing ingredients and drinking from, and straws are also smart buys.

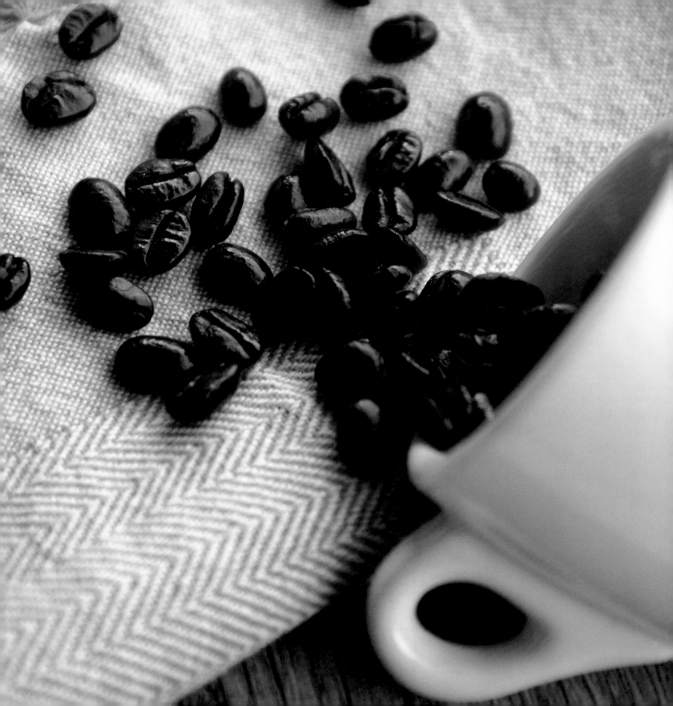

SUPERFOOD SMOOTHIE 101

Superfood smoothies are the star of the show. They can be complete meals that include all essential macro- and micronutrients, healthy versions of dessert-like smoothies we love to drink, and everything in between. My hope is that you will not only enjoy the recipes provided, but also use them as a starting point for your own concoctions. The following template will provide you with the means to do so.

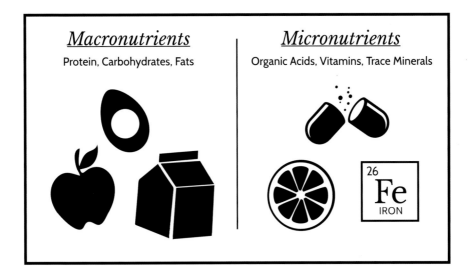

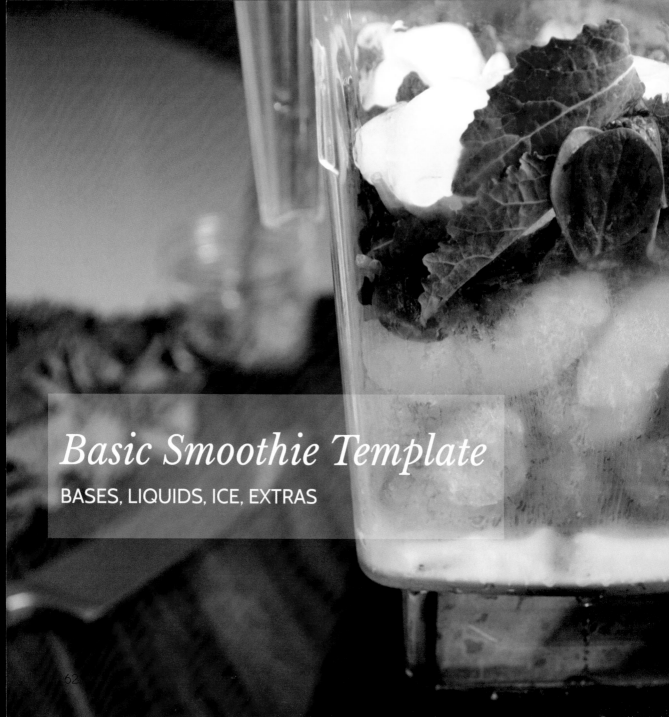

Basic Smoothie Template

BASES, LIQUIDS, ICE, EXTRAS

BASIC SMOOTHIE TEMPLATE

Most of the smoothies in this book follow the preceding template to achieve not only a healthy variety of nutrients, but also a suitable texture as well. Superfoods can be included in any of the following four categories. This is your guide for creating your own delicious recipes or for altering the recipes herein.

Bases: These are the main ingredients in the smoothie, and they usually provide the texture and thickness. This is a very broad category and can contain a wide variety of ingredients, such as whole soaked seeds, nuts, or fruits; fresh greens; fresh fruit; rolled oats; cooked brown rice; frozen fruit; and frozen vegetables.

Liquids: Most smoothies simply will not blend or will come out more like a pudding if you do not add liquid. Add more or less depending on your thickness preference. When adding pre-packaged liquids, be sure to avoid juices, as most have added sugar or have been pasteurized. Besides, you can usually add the fresh version of the whole fruit instead. Also, avoid sweetened varieties of seed and nut milks. Remember, we're trying to avoid added sugar. When possible, always go for fresh and homemade first. Liquids can include water, fresh coconut water, organic raw milk, fresh-squeezed citrus, cooled homemade tea, seed and nut milks, and freshly juiced hard vegetables (carrot, beet).

Ice: A thick smoothie will turn creamy, and a thin smoothie will become a frosty slushie with the addition of ice. It will also chill a smoothie (which is infinitely more palatable) that may have become slightly warm due to blending speed or the addition of warmer ingredients. Plain ice cubes work well, but water may down the flavors. You can also try many varieties of flavored ice, as mentioned in the Super-Flavored Ice chapter.

Extras: These are usually flavorings or sweeteners that may be needed to tone down the potency of certain ingredients, but can also include superfood powders and healthy fats. Examples include fruit powder, root powder, protein powder, spices, extracts, citrus zest, sea salt, honey, stevia, virgin coconut oil, and virgin olive oil.

Once you have chosen your ingredients from the four categories above, all that remains is adding them to your blender jar in such a way that minimizes *splashback* (like dumping frozen berries into liquid) and maximizes blending efficiency. To do so, always load in the following order:

1. Larger, harder **base** ingredients like frozen fruit, nuts, and grains. *If none exist, add ice first.*
2. Softer **base** ingredients like fresh fruit, greens, soaked nuts, seeds, and fruit.
3. All your **extras** like powders, spices, extracts, oils.
4. **Liquid**, then **ice**.

Give it all a gentle push down in the jar and blend away.

Blenders

These days, the selection of blenders on the market is varied, and almost all are suitable for superfood smoothies. I have used everything from a $40 Oster to a $500 Vitamix. As of this writing, I am currently in love with the Blendtec Total Blender and have used it successfully for the past four years.

These expensive, high-powered blenders like Vitamix and Blendtec do provide exceptional blending power and can pulverize just about anything you throw at, or *in*, them. The texture of your smoothies will certainly benefit from making an investment in that direction. However, they are not necessary for any recipes in this book.

Ninja makes a blender that is significantly cheaper and Nutri Bullet makes a compact, on-the-go blender at the same affordable price point (about $100). Oster and Hamilton Beach make blenders that are even more affordable at around $50. Although they don't blend ingredients quite as smooth as the high-powered blenders, they are a suitable substitute. Remember, the important part is to build a habit of making and consuming superfood drinks, so don't stress over the blender until that habit is set and you can afford to perfect your approach.

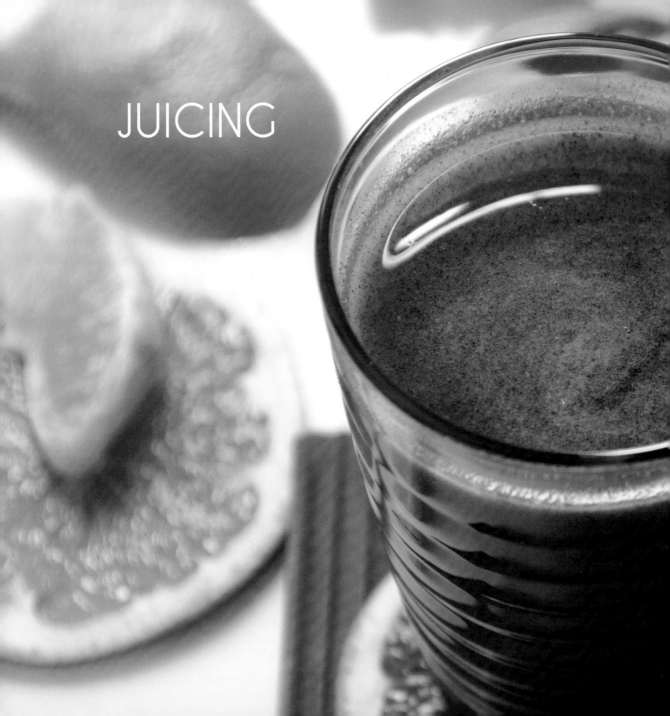

JUICING

SUPERFOOD JUICING 101

Juicing is infinitely simpler than creating a palatable smoothie. Since we're not working with textures—it's just juice—we have no need for layering or separating ingredient types into categories. Instead we have vegetable juice, fruit juice, or more likely some combination of both. While some recipes in this book follow that very simple outline, to make things interesting, there are quite a few that require a blender to add superfood powders and/or super-flavored ice. These additions can of course be removed, and you can enjoy the juice on its own just as well.

It is best to gather all your ingredients, chop them into manageable pieces, and put them in a bowl by the juicer before you begin. Once juiced, give the glass a stir or add some ice and enjoy. Simple as that.

For the recipes that require adding powders or other ingredients, I like to add the other ingredient to the blender first, pour the fresh juice on top, and let it sit for a minute or two, then blend. If the drink becomes too frothy, add ice to balance.

Remember, it's very difficult to go wrong with mixing juices. Experiment with ingredients to find new flavors to love.

Juicers

There are three categories of juicers, each with different price points, yields, and nutrient value. The recipes in this book were made using a Breville Ikon centrifugal juicer, so ingredient quantities may need to be slightly adjusted based on the type of juicer you own.

Centrifugal: This is the most common and most affordable of the three—usually in the $80 to $200 realm. Fruits and vegetables are grated against a fast-spinning blade with the juice flowing through a mesh filter and the pulp separated into a separate receptacle. These produce the lowest yields, will not juice small leafy items like wheatgrass, and may have trouble even with larger green, leafy vegetables. They also yield a juice with heavy foam because of the fast speeds. Almost all department store juicers are of the centrifugal type.

Masticating *(single-gear)*: These juicers operate at slower speeds than centrifugal juicers and use a single gear or auger to grind and chew fruits and vegetables, thereby extracting much more juice and nutrients. Most have no problem with wheatgrass and other green, leafy vegetables and yield a juice with no foam. They are generally priced from $200 to $300.

Triturating *(twin-gear)*: These work similarly to masticating juicers, except they have two gears or augers instead of one and operate at even slower speeds. You get the most juice and nutrient yields possible from every type of fruit and vegetable. They are without a doubt the best type of juicer to own, and the price reflects that. They run anywhere from $400 to upwards of $1000.

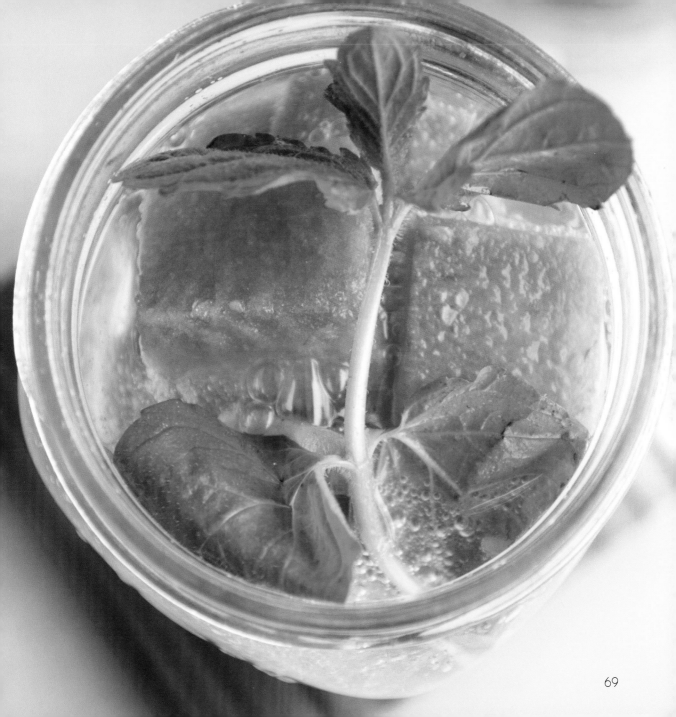

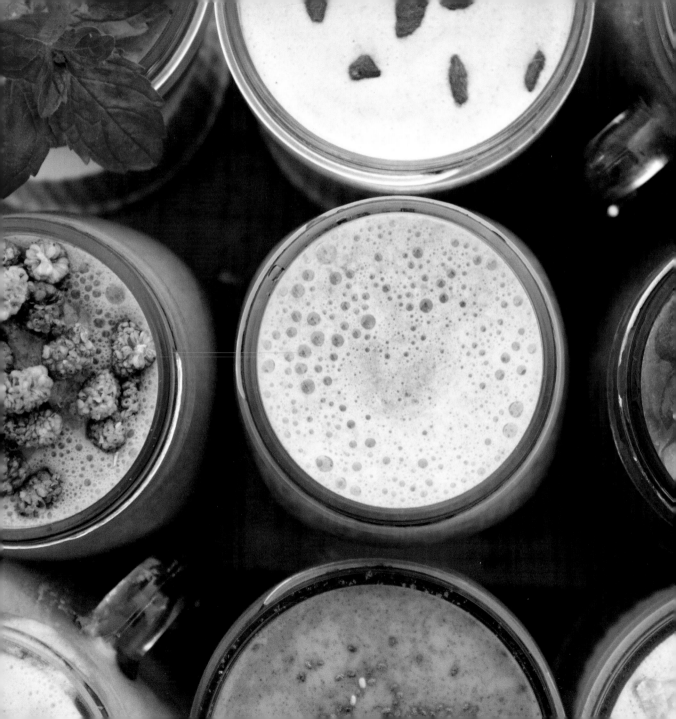

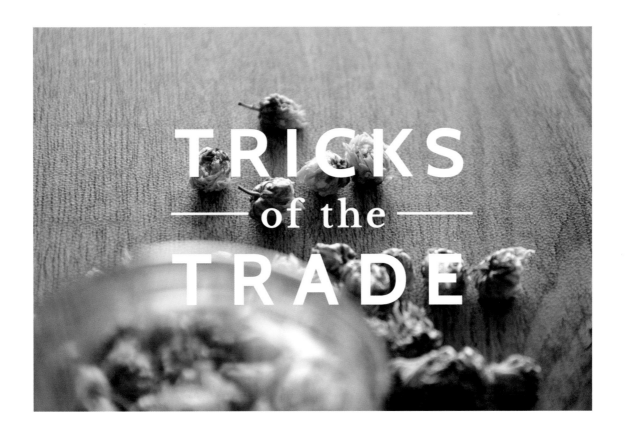

TRICKS —— of the —— TRADE

Throughout the years, I have refined my superfood drink techniques in terms of cost effectiveness, palatable textures, and overall efficiency. The following is the best of those refinements.

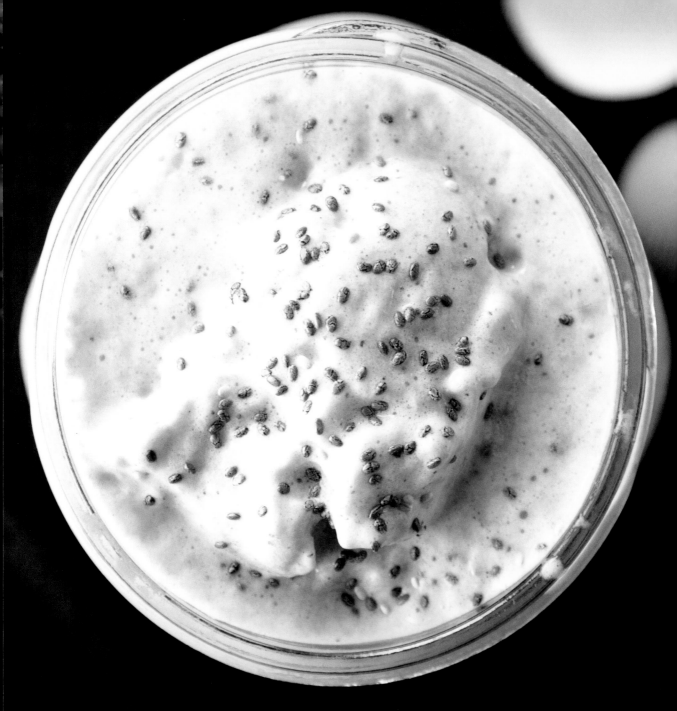

THAT CREAMY TEXTURE

Some smoothies can foam or separate due to an overload of ingredients containing insoluble fiber. The best way to fix that is to add ingredients with soluble fiber. This also gives the smoothie a palatable creaminess. These ingredients include: avocado, banana, mango, milk (coconut and organic raw), organic whole milk yogurt, cooked grains (brown rice and rolled oats), soaked nuts, and seeds.

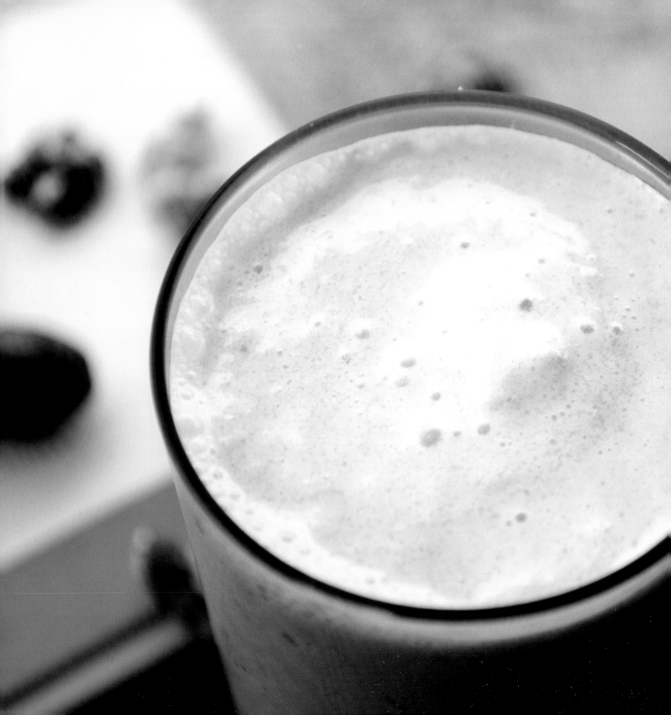

SMOOTHIES: STIRRED, NOT BLENDED

Milk almost always works best when stirred in after the bulk of the smoothie has been blended, otherwise you'll end up with a huge head of froth on your smoothie; slightly reminiscent of the less healthy drink you'd get at a local pub. The exception is when the recipe doesn't call for any other liquid besides milk. In that instance, it's best to add only enough milk to get the ingredients to blend, then stir in the rest.

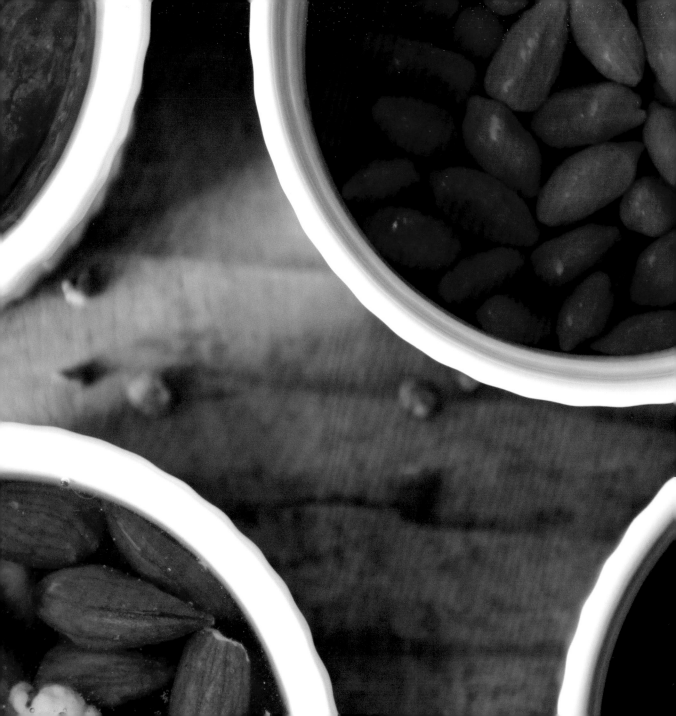

SOAKING DRIED FRUIT, NUTS & SEEDS

There are two reasons to pre-soak dried fruit, nuts, and seeds: 1) it enhances the digestibility, and 2) while high-powered blenders like Vitamix and Blendtec can blend hard ingredients without issue, those with inexpensive blenders will benefit significantly from softening the fruit, nuts, and seeds first.

Nuts & Seeds: Add the nuts or seeds to a small container or mason jar, leaving enough room to add twice as much water. Let soak for a minimum of two hours and up to twenty-four hours, periodically rinsing and replacing the water.

Dried Fruit: Use the desired amount of fruit in the recipe, along with the amount of liquid called for in that same recipe (water, coconut water, etc.). Let soak in a container for twenty to thirty minutes. The fruit will noticeably plump. Use the fruit and the soaking liquid when ready.

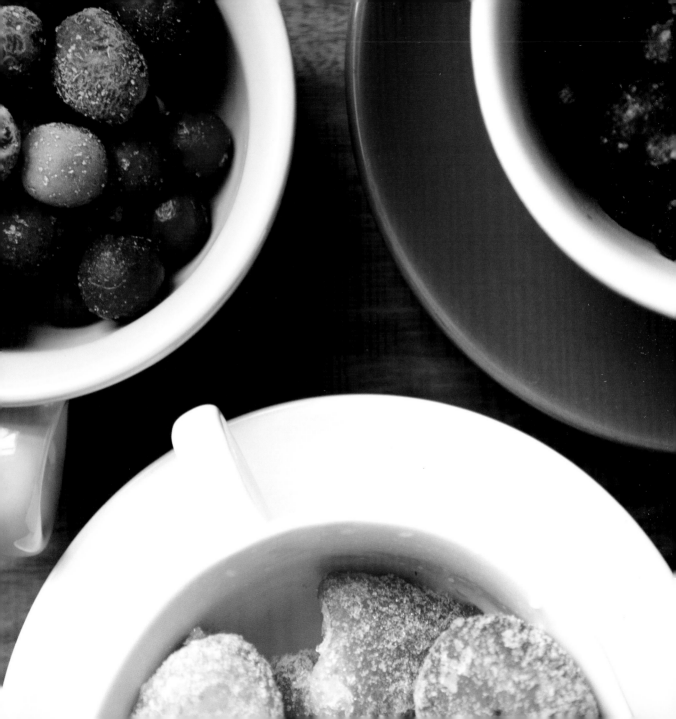

FROZEN FRUITS & VEGETABLES

Not only are frozen foods more cost effective than their fresh counterparts, but they last significantly longer. They also have the added benefit of muting certain flavors, like broccoli, and replacing ice cubes to chill a smoothie. My favorite frozen fruits and vegetables found in almost all markets are blueberries, strawberries, mangoes, broccoli, and spinach.

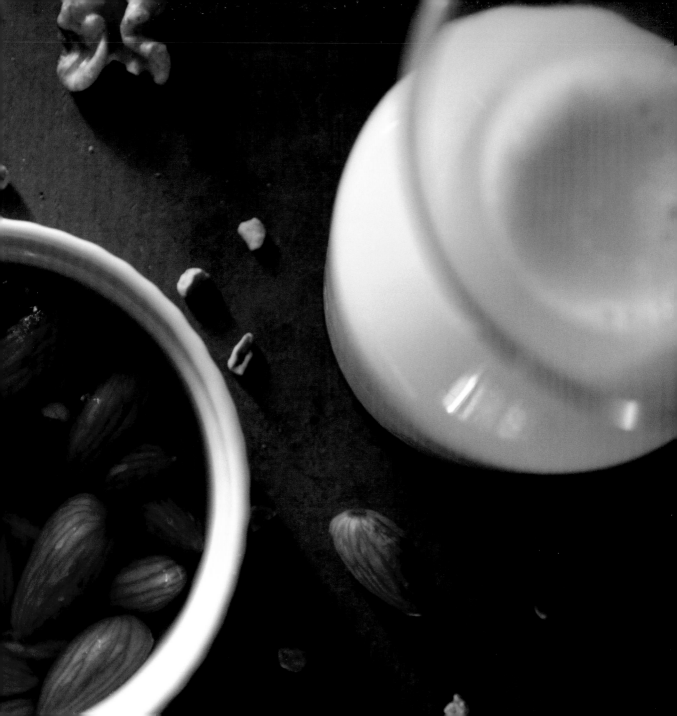

NUT & SEED MILKS

This is much easier than most people realize. All you need are three things: a blender (which you should already have), your ingredients (whatever seeds or nuts you want to use, and any optional flavorings), and some sort of strainer, sieve, or cheesecloth (they even make nut milk bags). The process is quite simple:

1. Pre-soak your nuts or seeds (½ cup) for 2–8 hours in water (until they are plump). Then rinse thoroughly.
2. Add the nuts or seeds to your blender with about 2¾ cups of fresh water (more for a thinner milk and less for more of a cream). Optional: add flavorings like vanilla bean or extract, cacao powder, cinnamon, or stevia.
3. Blend until smooth and creamy (about 1–2 minutes).
4. Strain and store the liquid in a sealed mason jar in the refrigerator for up to a week.

Much more affordable, healthier, and tastier than store-bought seed and nut milks. Try almonds, cashews, macadamias, hemp seeds, sunflower seeds, and more.

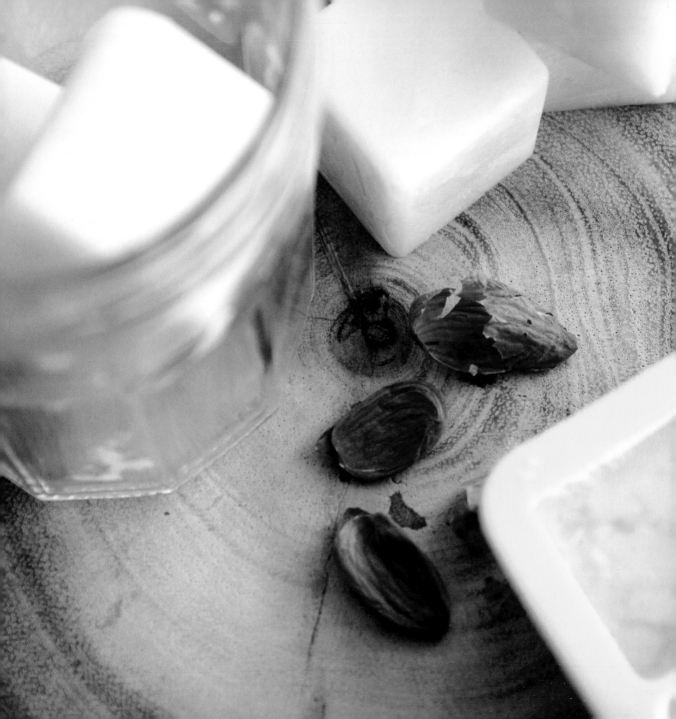

SUPER-FLAVORED ICE

Upgrade your superfood drinks by making your own super-ice! Just add herbs, fruit, milks, or teas to your ice cube trays. Some of my favorites are: almond milk, green tea, coconut water, mint and blueberries with water, and strawberry and basil with water. This is a great alternative to adding unhealthy, sugar-laden ice creams or plain old ice. Silicone ice cube trays work best, but be sure to cover with plastic wrap or tray tops to minimize odor absorption.

SIMPLE SUBSTITUTIONS

We don't always have access to the more exotic superfood ingredients, or perhaps we've just run out. Whatever the reason, the following ingredients can be used interchangeably without deviating too much from the original flavor, texture, and nutrient makeup:

- Dates, raisins, mulberries
- Raw milk, almond milk, coconut milk, hemp milk, etc.
- Açaí (powder), maqui (powder), camu camu (powder), blackberries, blueberries, strawberries, raspberries
- Pomegranate seeds, cranberries
- Cacao, cocoa (sugar-free)
- Flaxseed, chia seeds, hemp seeds
- Spirulina, chlorella, wheatgrass
- Brown rice, rolled oats
- Maca powder, protein powder
- Almonds, walnuts
- Kale, chard, spinach, lettuce
- Arugula, watercress

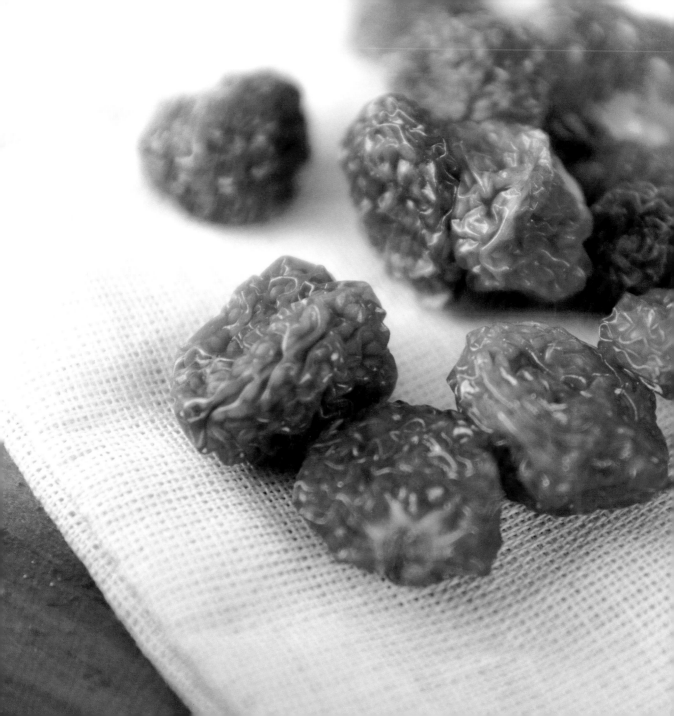

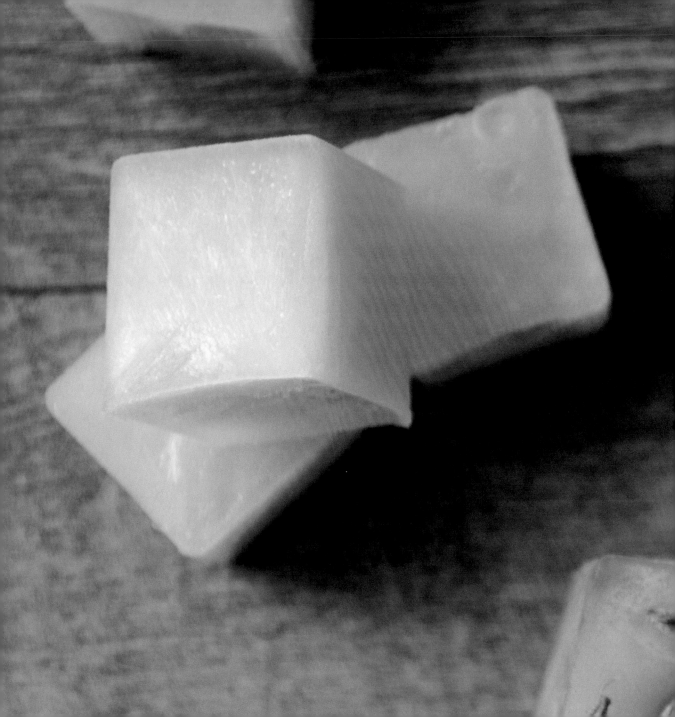

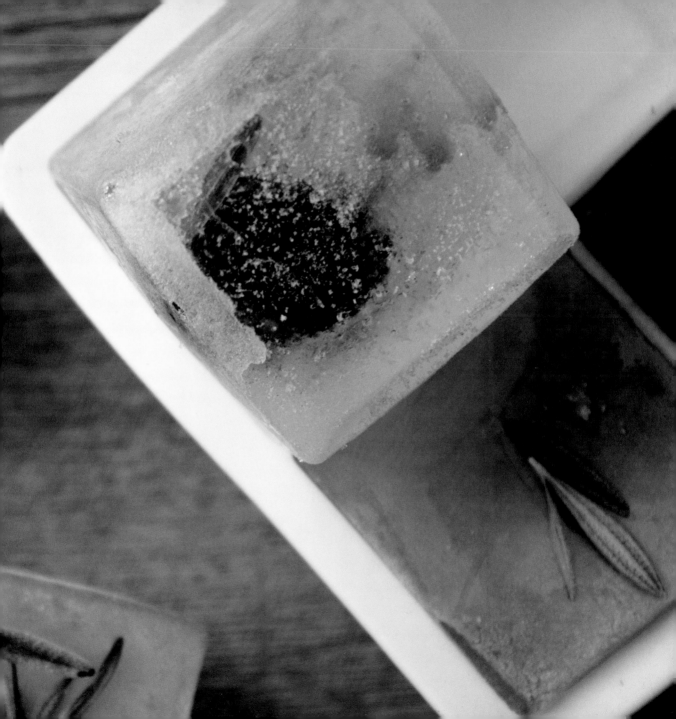

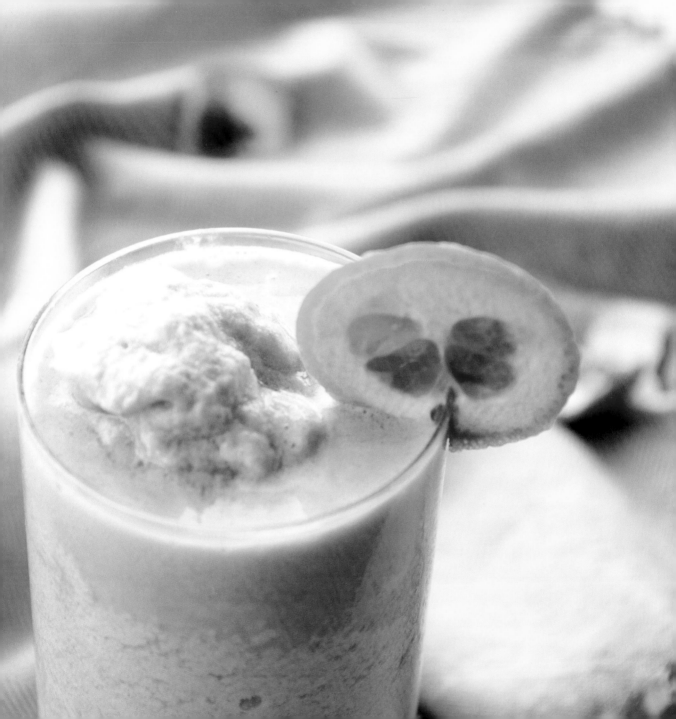

THE DIET

When most people make reference to a *diet*, they are usually speaking more specifically of *dietary habits*; ones that they are more than likely considering changing to accomplish a specific goal. Weight loss, weight gain, to cleanse the body of previously poor dietary choices, to avoid or cure some sort of ailment, etc. It is reactionary rather than consistent and this, I believe, is where we go wrong with regard to our nutrition and, ultimately, our wellbeing. These re-action-based diets, or **ReDiets**, to coin a phrase, are no doubt useful, but they generally represent a backward motion. The prefix *re-* indicates a return to a previous condition—restoration—and works quite well here. They are meant to get you back on track with your regular or *true* diet.

Your true diet is the food you consume on a regular basis. Simple as that. Superfood drinks are meant to fit in neatly with your true diet as a way to quickly and efficiently supply the body with a good amount of the proper nutrition it requires. Adding them is as easy as making the decision to do so. Superfood drinks work wonderfully as a breakfast or pre-breakfast, depending on your caloric requirements, as well as snacks throughout the day when needed.

Aside from supplying your body with high-quality macro- and micronutrients, superfood drinks have another strong benefit to making them part of your regular diet—they suppress the urge to overeat. If our bodies are truly satiated, in that they are getting what they require to function at peak efficiency, those hunger pangs go away and the urge to stuff ourselves with low-quality empty calories slowly diminishes over time. That isn't to say that your *cravings* for chocolate chip cookies will evaporate overnight—there are psychological hang-ups involved as well—but it does make it measurably easier.

However, since there are certainly times when *rediets* can be helpful, superfood drinks lend themselves quite well to the following:

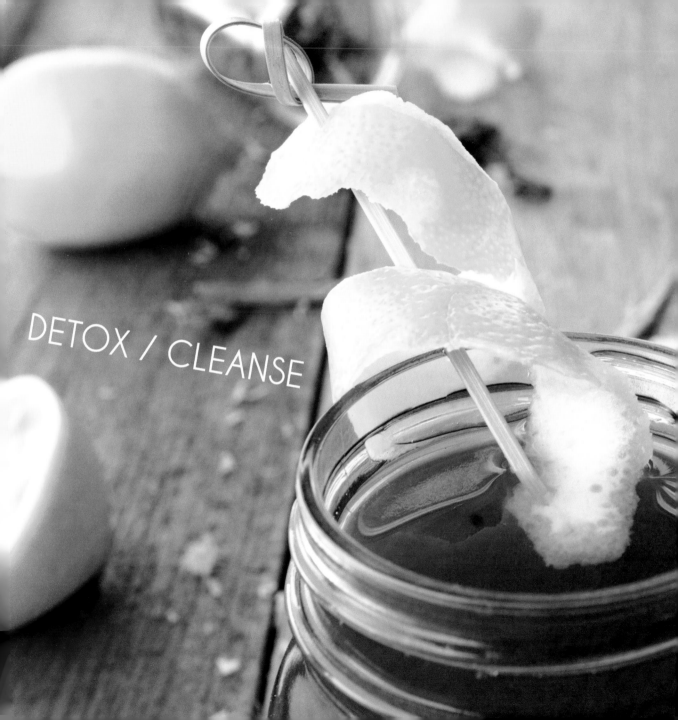

DETOX / CLEANSE

DETOX/CLEANSE

Typically, detoxing or cleansing diets have you eating well below your required daily calories for a series of days; essentially fasting between tiny meals. While fasting and calorie restriction can certainly be beneficial to your health, it isn't recommended to do so for longer than 8–16 hours. Otherwise, you're just denying your body the important nutrients it needs to function. Instead, we're going to focus on using superfood drinks as the base of our meals. This way we get all the macro- and micronutrients our system needs while still maintaining a semi-fasting and calorie-restricted state. Using superfood drinks also provides most of what is needed to support the organs your body naturally uses to flush itself of toxins. These organs are:

- the **liver**, which is your system's first and main toxin filter.
- the **colon**, which contains bacteria that help flush toxins via defecation.
- the **kidneys**, which filter blood and help remove toxins via urination.

Foods that support the liver include: high antioxidant fruits like berries, green tea, apples, dark leafy greens, cruciferous vegetables, lemons, turmeric, beets, and carrots.

Foods that support the colon include: water, fiber (from fruits and vegetables), probiotic and fermented foods like yogurt, pickles, kimchi, miso, and sauerkraut.

Foods that support the kidneys include: water, cruciferous vegetables, and berries.

Combining a superfood smoothie, juice, and plenty of infused water through-out the day with supplemental colon supporting foods like miso and sauerkraut makes for the perfect detox/cleanse diet. Choose different drinks every day for no more than 2–3 days for the perfect toxin-flushing experience. Then slowly return to your regular diet, with hopefully fewer artificial foods this time, while keeping a superfood drink or two in your daily routine.

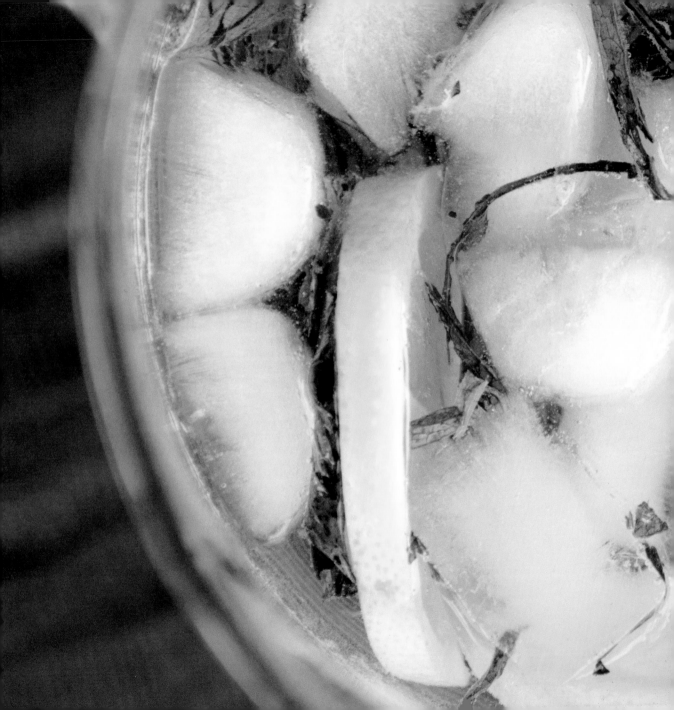

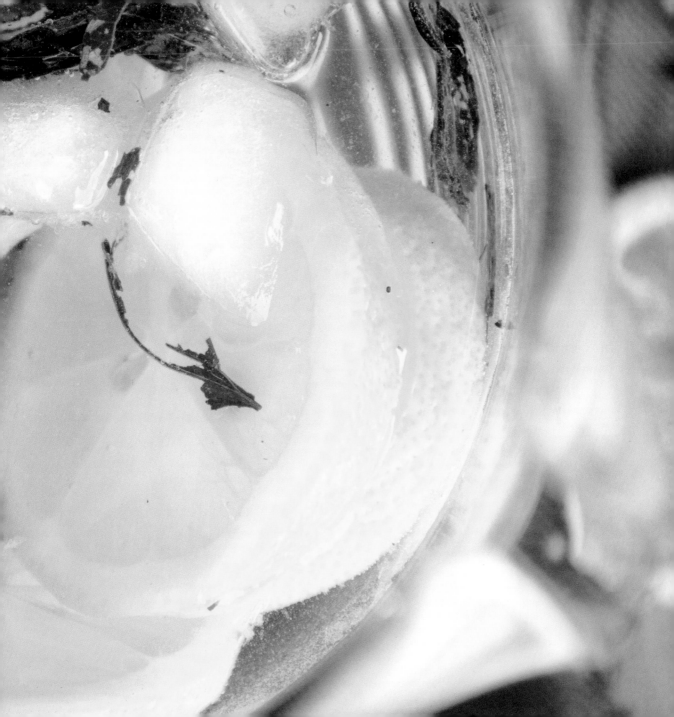

WEIGHT LOSS/GAIN

There are no specific foods, pills, or shortcuts to losing excess weight. In fact, there are essentially three ways to effectively lose and/or maintain weight, and all three contain varying degrees of diet *and* exercise:

1. Very low-calorie diet with little to no exercise
2. Very high-calorie diet with an extreme level of exercise
3. A balance of the two. The *Goldilocks* of weight management.

These are simplified, of course, since everybody is different and certain medical conditions have not been considered, but in general, these are the rules of the game. We'll dig in a little deeper to better understand what they mean and how superfood drinks fit in.

The low-calorie, no exercise plan will keep most people at a low weight but is still considered to be unhealthy because it puts your body in a situation that is prone to atrophy. I know a great many people who want to lose weight but despise exercise—an unfortunate pairing. I would argue that a better, tighter goal would be to become a healthier person. Manageable weight, and indeed weight loss, is a byproduct of that goal, as well as gaining increased energy, vitality, mental acuity, etc. Simply reducing calorie intake while remaining docile can certainly shed pounds, and you'll be better off than you were with the excess weight, but why sell yourself short? This is your body, the vehicle of your mind, your thoughts, desires, dreams. Treat it with the respect it—*you*—deserve.

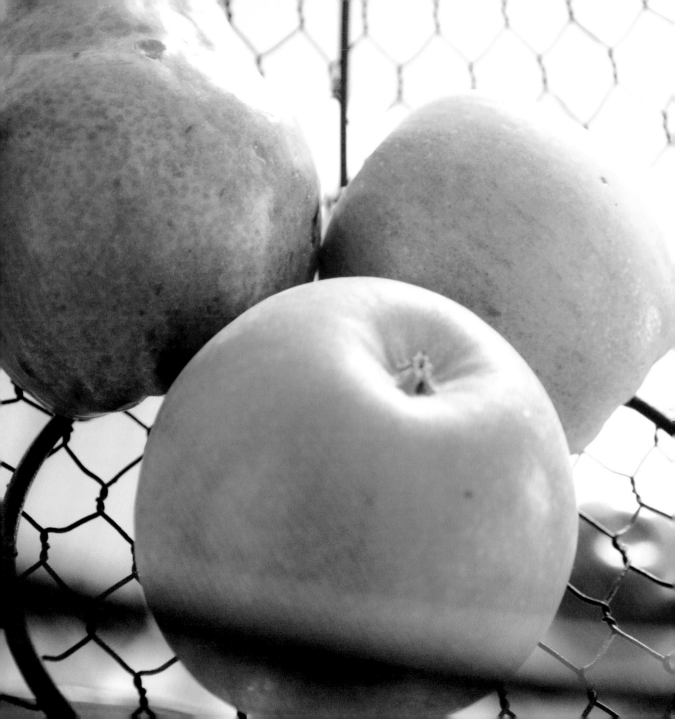

The high-calorie, extreme exercise option is mostly targeted toward athletes and will keep them at a pretty level weight depending on how far along they are in their training or sport and in which direction they tip the diet/exercise scale. Weight gain certainly exists at this level, in the form of increased muscle mass depending on the type of exercises performed; for instance, a strength-training program as opposed to marathon training.

The balanced plan is what most people should strive for and is our primary focus with regard to superfood drinks. Those who could do with a bit more weight on their bones can use superfood drinks as a supplement to their regular meals. High-protein options work wonderfully as post-workout meals and provide the body with what it needs to repair and grow. For those wishing to lose weight, adding superfood drinks as a meal replacement or a pre-meal can work wonders for providing necessary nutrients, thereby satiating the body and allowing for less overeating. Couple this with regular exercise and you'll be well on your way to a healthier, more manageable weight.

In this way, the weight loss/gain diet starts as a *rediet* and eventually becomes just another aspect to your *true* diet. Just the way it should be.

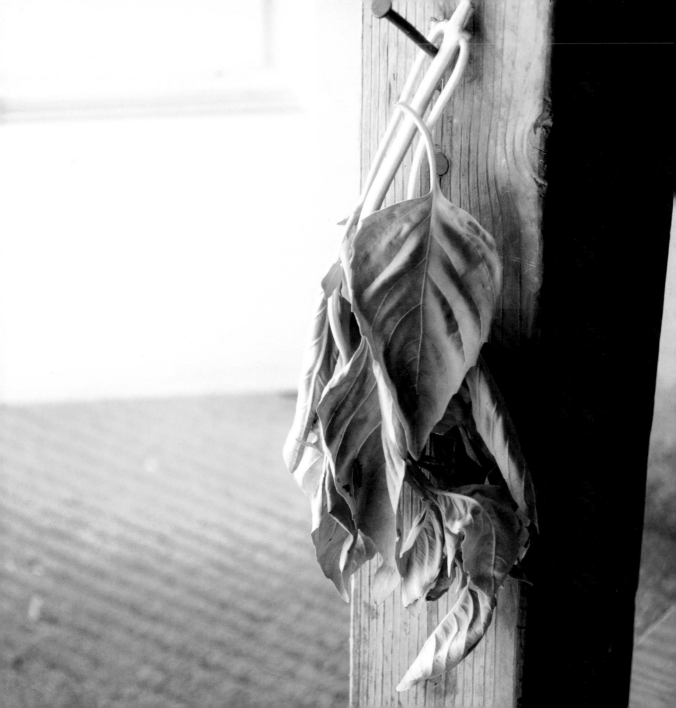

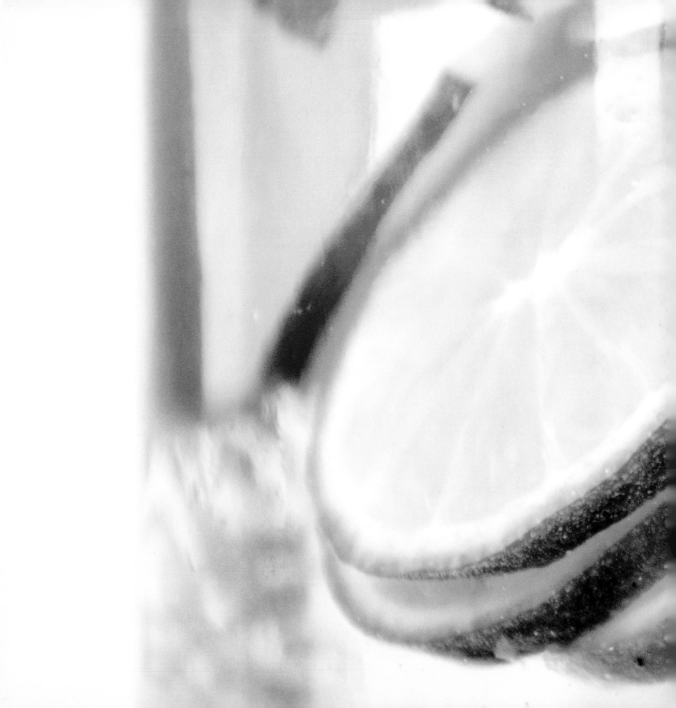

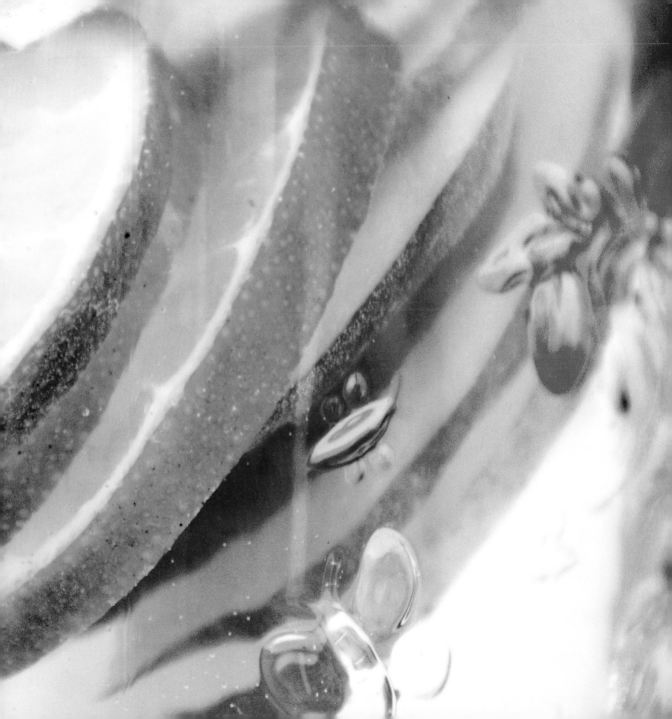

RECIPES

The following recipes have been separated into four sections: smoothies, juices, infused waters, and coffees, teas, and other drinks. Most recipe pages have a *personal touch* area that can be used for notes and ingredient changes; feel free to experiment with ingredients as you see fit. The following tips will help you get the best out of your superfood drinks:

- When blending and juicing fruits and vegetables with green tops like strawberries and carrots, don't remove them—they're nutritious!
- Always used unsweetened milks, powders, and fruits when buying from the market.
- Remember, we're working with fruits and vegetables with varying flavors and sizes throughout the year, so color, texture, and flavors will vary. Don't hesitate to adjust for these differences.
- Is your smoothie foamy or separating? Consider adding banana, mango, avocado, milks, or ice to fix.
- Add ice for a more frosty or ice cream–like texture, and liquid to thin the drink out.
- Add sweeteners (listed in the Ingredients section) if the drink isn't sweet enough for you.
- If the drink is too sweet, consider adding water, ice, or other non-sweet ingredients.
- When adding egg to hot liquid, do so slowly while the blender is running to avoid cooking.

BENEFITS LEGEND

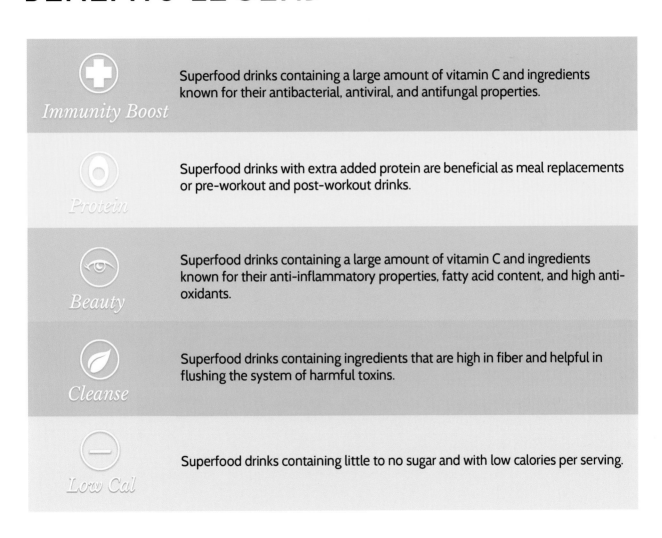

Immunity Boost
Superfood drinks containing a large amount of vitamin C and ingredients known for their antibacterial, antiviral, and antifungal properties.

Protein
Superfood drinks with extra added protein are beneficial as meal replacements or pre-workout and post-workout drinks.

Beauty
Superfood drinks containing a large amount of vitamin C and ingredients known for their anti-inflammatory properties, fatty acid content, and high anti-oxidants.

Cleanse
Superfood drinks containing ingredients that are high in fiber and helpful in flushing the system of harmful toxins.

Low Cal
Superfood drinks containing little to no sugar and with low calories per serving.

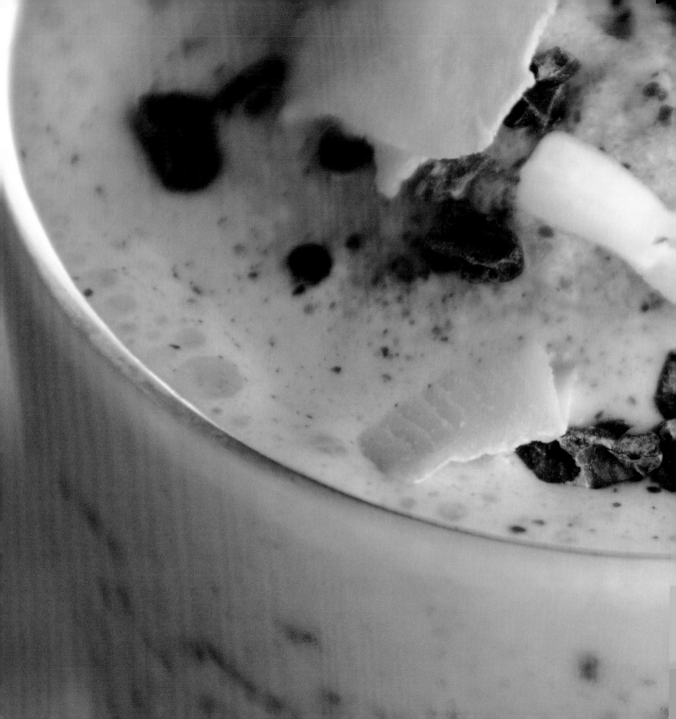

SMOOTHIES

Superfood smoothies are the most comprehensive superfood drinks in this book. Not only do they contain vitamins and minerals from fresh fruits and vegetables, but they also retain the fiber and often include highly nutritious fats. Macro- and micronutrient complete.

Components of Smoothies

BASE, LIQUIDS, ICE, EXTRAS

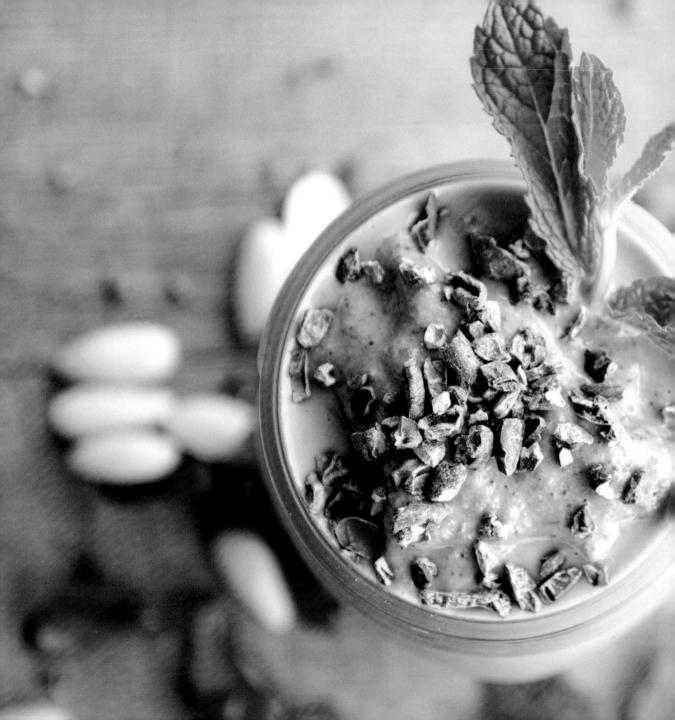

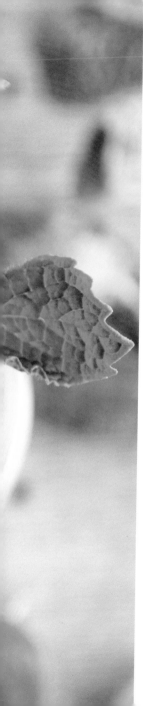

CHOCOLATE MINT
Makes three 16-oz. servings

4 pitted dates

1–2 cups raw milk (or almond milk)

¼ cup soaked almonds

2 tbsp. cacao nibs

½ cup packed mint leaves

½ small avocado

2 cups coconut ice

Chocolate and mint together provide a tasty treat that never fails to satisfy. Reminiscent of cookie and candy standards, Chocolate Mint pays homage to some nostalgic favorites. With this creamy drink, you can enjoy the combination guilt-free with the added bonus that it is actually good for you!

Skin all soaked almonds before placing them and the rest of the ingredients in a blender to blend to a chunky minty goodness.

Personal Touch:

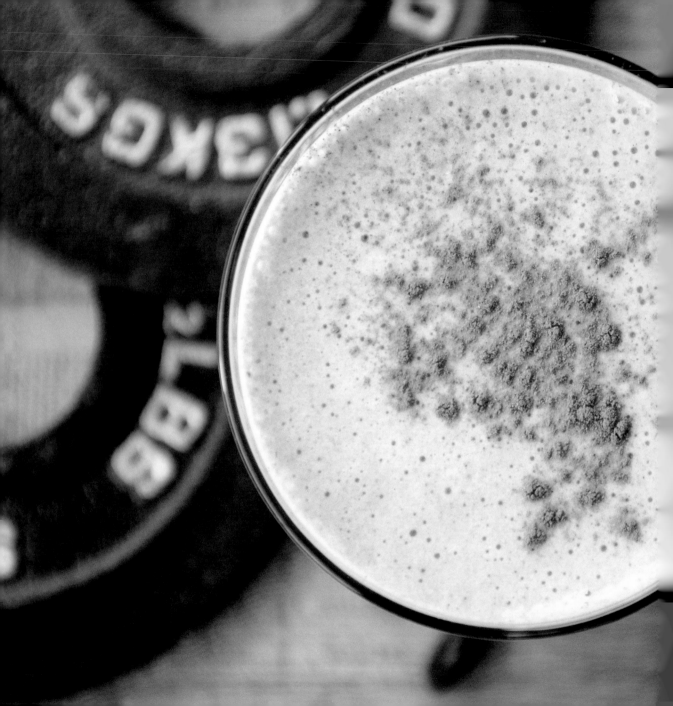

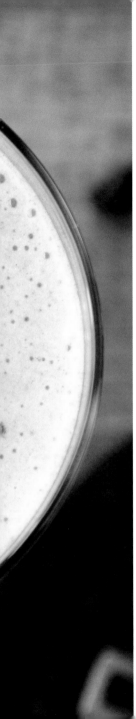

PERFECT POST-WORKOUT

Makes one 22-oz. serving

1 cup cooked organic brown rice (cold)

or ½ cup uncooked organic rolled oats

3–4 tbsp. organic raisins

1–2 scoops of high-quality protein powder

1 tsp. cinnamon

2 tsp. maca powder

1 cup water

1 cup organic raw whole milk

After a serious workout where you've depleted your energy stores, it's important that you refuel your body to recover and get stronger so that you can meet your next personal record. Combining healthy carbs like rolled oats or organic rice with protein powder and natural sugar from raisins provides the substance you need to avoid muscle depletion and backsliding from your fitness progress.

Combine all ingredients in a blender and blend until creamy.

Personal Touch:

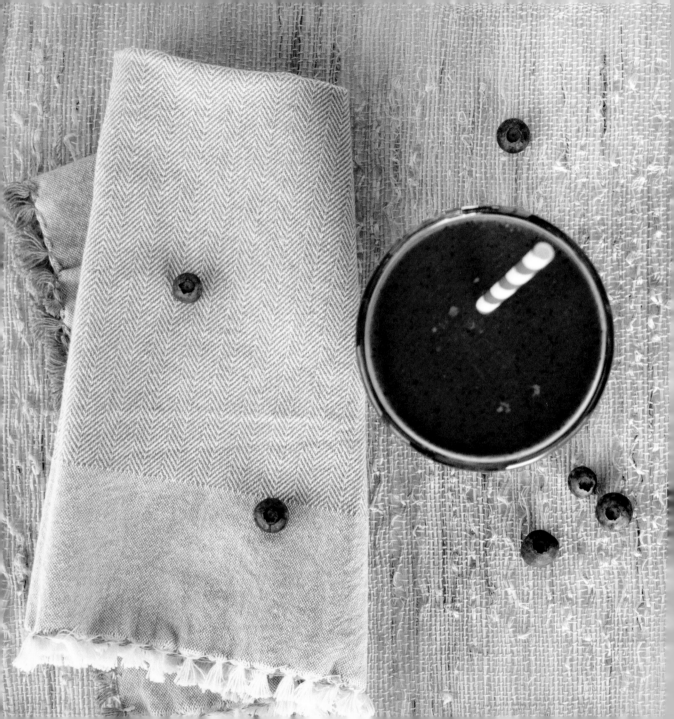

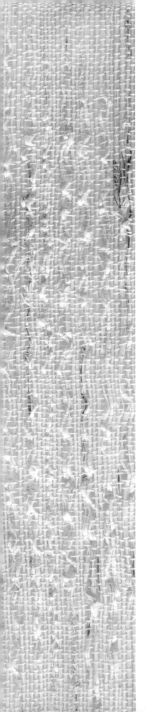

HELLO WORLD
Makes two 16-oz. servings

1 cup fresh or frozen organic blueberries

2 big handfuls of organic greens (whatever you have on-hand)

1 small banana

½ avocado

1 tsp. matcha

1 cup water

1 almond ice

1 cup organic raw whole milk

The perfect introduction to the language of green drinks. A quick look at the source code of this drink and you'll be surprised that its creamy blueberry goodness delivers such great flavor and nutrition. The energy surge will have you coding Hello World every morning.

Compile. Execute.

Personal Touch: _____

_____

_____

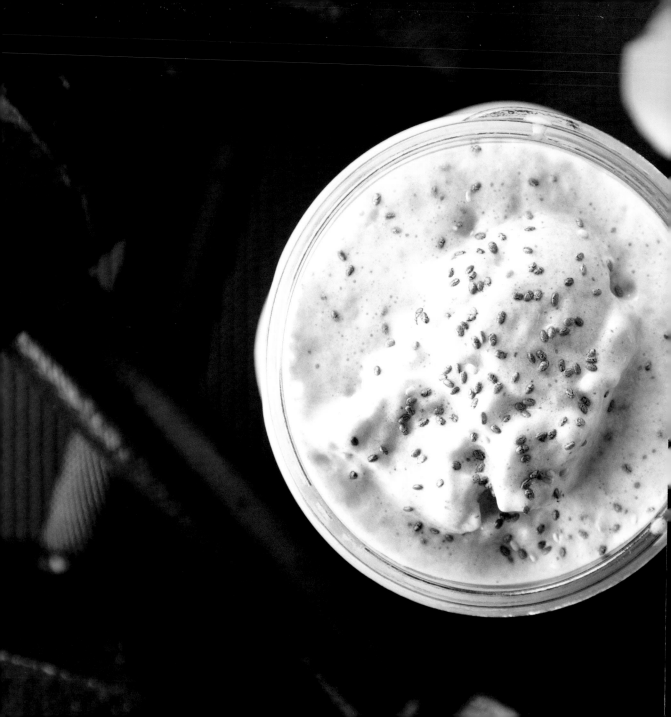

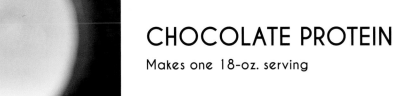

CHOCOLATE PROTEIN

Makes one 18-oz. serving

1–2 scoops protein powder (chocolate or vanilla)

2–3 raw organic pastured egg yolks

2 tsp. lemon juice

1 tbsp. cacao powder

1 tbsp. chia seeds

1 cup water

1 cup ice

After a satisfying workout, it's hard to not just give in and go to the frozen yogurt shop. This post-workout protein powerhouse has everything you need to recover, plus such sweet dessert flavors that you'll be hitting the gym just so you can run home to blend this baby up and drink it down.

Combine all ingredients together in a blender and mix until frothy.

Personal Touch:

TROPICAL STORM

Makes two 18-oz. servings

juice of 2 large carrots

1 cup frozen mango

1 cup frozen pineapple

2 collard green leaves (stemmed)

5 large basil leaves

6 mint leaves

¼ jalapeño

This great combination provides some fabulous tropical tastes that pack a real healthy punch with a kick of jalapeño. This is sure to get your circulation moving.

Juice carrots separately. Blend all ingredients together and serve up in a tall glass with a straw.

Change it up: Kale and collard greens are often exchangeable. If you have a preference, both options work well with the fruit pairing above.

Personal Touch:

CAPT. DR. KALE

Makes two 16-oz. servings

1 cup coffee

2 cups of baby kale

2 tbsp. cacao nibs

¾ cup almond milk

1 scoop whey protein powder

1 banana

1 large date

"Life is short, eat dessert first!" For our intrepid Capt. Dr. Caela, rounds at the hospital never stop, so it's hard to know when dessert ends and breakfast begins. This shake gives her all the energy and nutrients she needs to keep going shift after shift, so she can drink to your health as well as her own. On the chance you miss your opportunity for your daily intake of greens in each meal, there's always dessert.

Brew up one cup of coffee. Combine coffee and all ingredients into blender and blend until smooth.

Personal Touch:

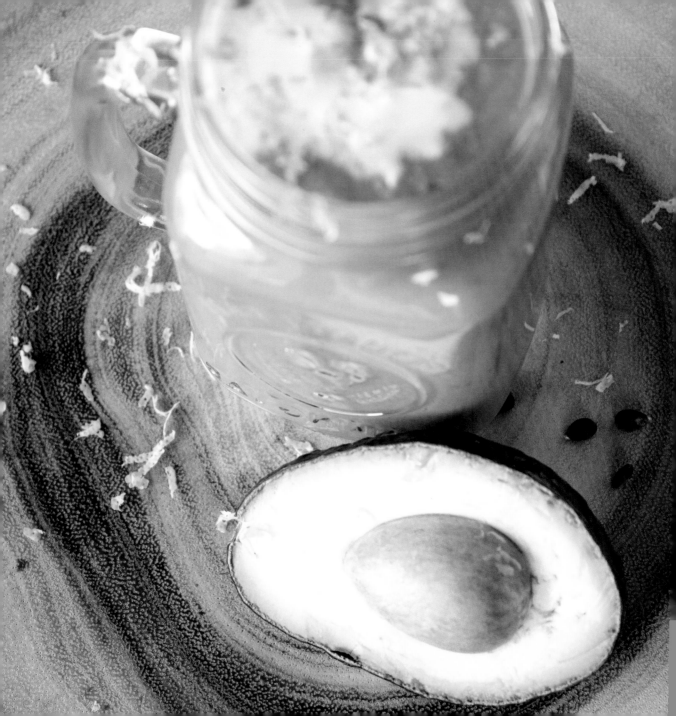

APPLE CREAM

Makes two 18-oz. servings

2 handfuls organic spinach

1 organic apple (peeled and cored)

½ avocado

2 tsp. spirulina

½ lemon (juice)

½ cup coconut milk

1 cup water

1–2 cups ice

Popeye would approve of this flavorful combination of apple, avocado, and spinach, as it is also a power booster with the added help of spirulina, which contains higher protein levels than red meat. This creamy concoction packs a healthy punch of flavor!

Place all ingredients in a high-powered blender and blend. If your blender runs under 1000 watts, juice apple first or cut into smaller pieces. Blend until creamy and smooth. Serve with a straw.

Personal Touch:

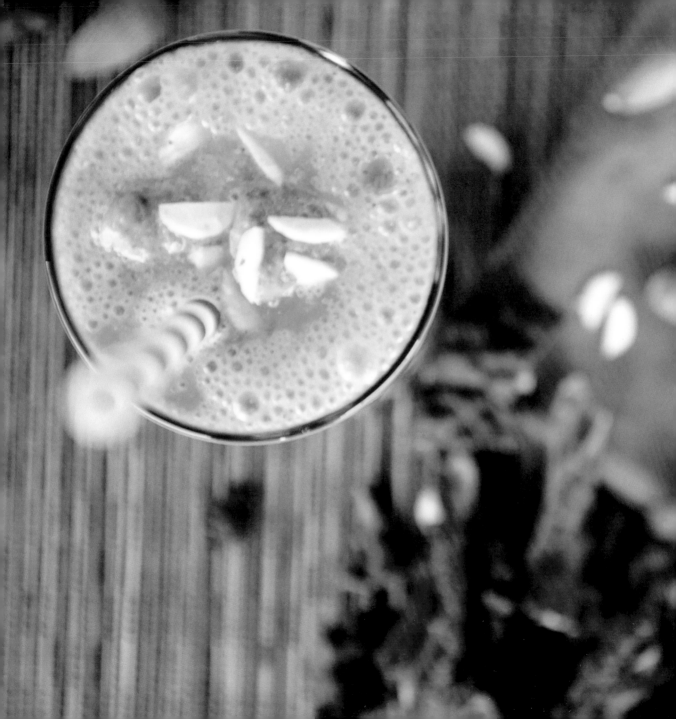

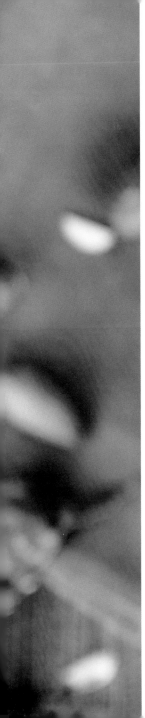

GREEN ALMOND

Makes one 16-oz. serving

1–2 handfuls organic kale
1 small banana
1 tbsp. almond butter
1 cup water
2 cups almond ice

This drink is loaded with nutrients and is a real palate pleaser. The combination of sweet bananas and almond flavor blend with the kale to make a fresh superfood smoothie.

Blend together all ingredients with a high powered blender until creamy. Serve immediately.

Personal Touch:

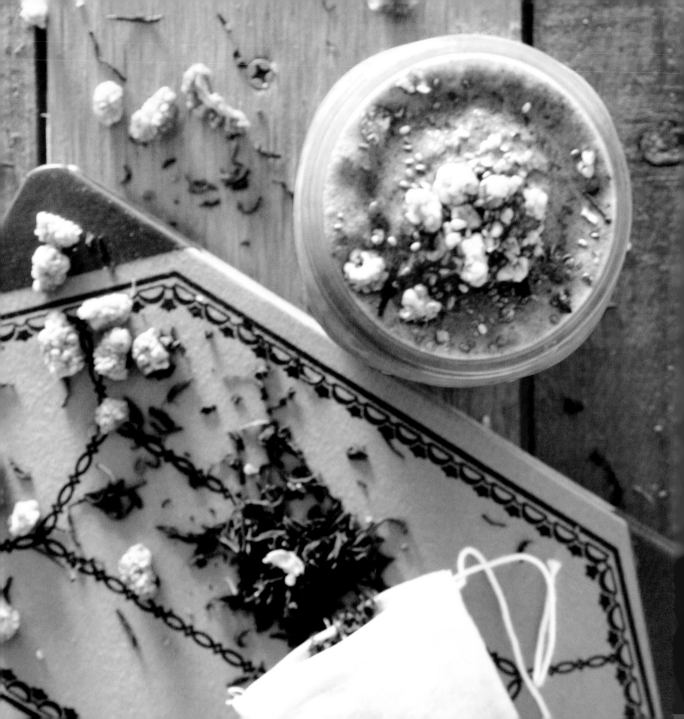

BLUE CHAI CRUNCH

Makes two 18-oz. servings

1 cup fresh or frozen organic blueberries

1 cup açaí berries (frozen) or 1 tbsp. powder

1 tbsp. chai tea (powder)

2–3 tbsp. chia seeds

1 tsp. vanilla extract

2 cups organic raw whole milk or almond milk

1 tbsp. dried mulberries on top

The wonderful crunchy texture of the dried mulberry topping on this smoothie adds rustic appeal as well as flavor. The ingredients like açaí berries compound the flavors as well as provide the benefits of disease-fighting antioxidants. This delectable drink will be enjoyed in all its chewy goodness.

Add all ingredients except dried mulberries to blender and blend until smooth. Top with dried mulberries.

Personal Touch:

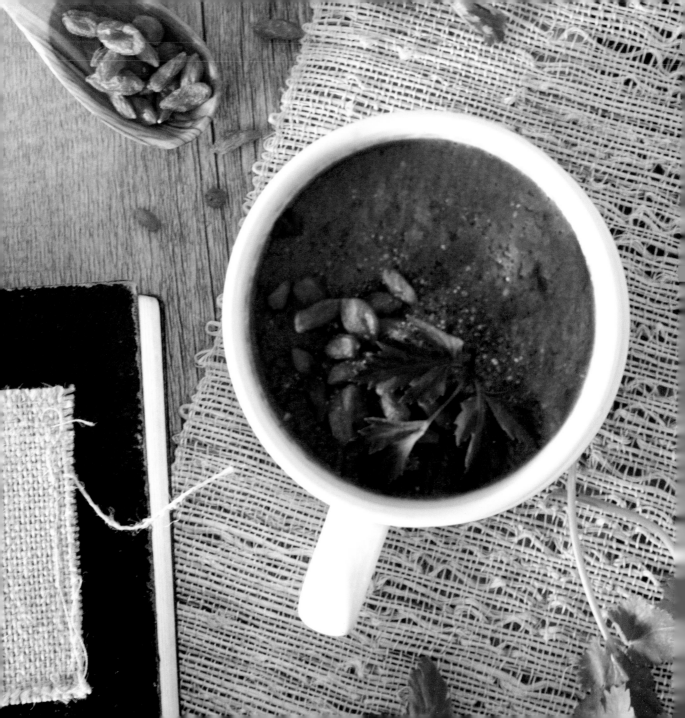

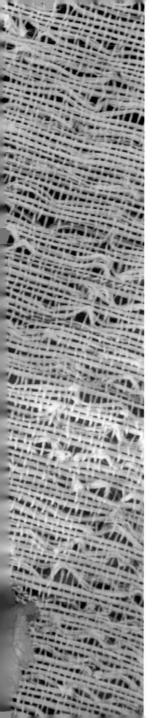

SOUP TO GOJI
Makes two 16-oz. servings

2 organic roma tomatoes

1 handful organic parsley

1 handful organic cilantro

1 small organic cucumber (peeled)

1 clove garlic

1–2 tbsp. goji berries

½ lemon (juice)

½ cup water

2 tbsp. extra virgin olive oil

salt, pepper, and cayenne to taste

Our play on a savory summer soup favorite, Soup To Goji adds a sour spicy element to the rustic Italian flavors of a classic gazpacho. Goji berries are great additions to many savory snacks.

Place all ingredients, save for the oil, into a high-powered blender or food processor. After initially blended, pulse the blender while drizzling in the oil. Serve in bowl or large cappuccino mug with a spoon.

Personal Touch:

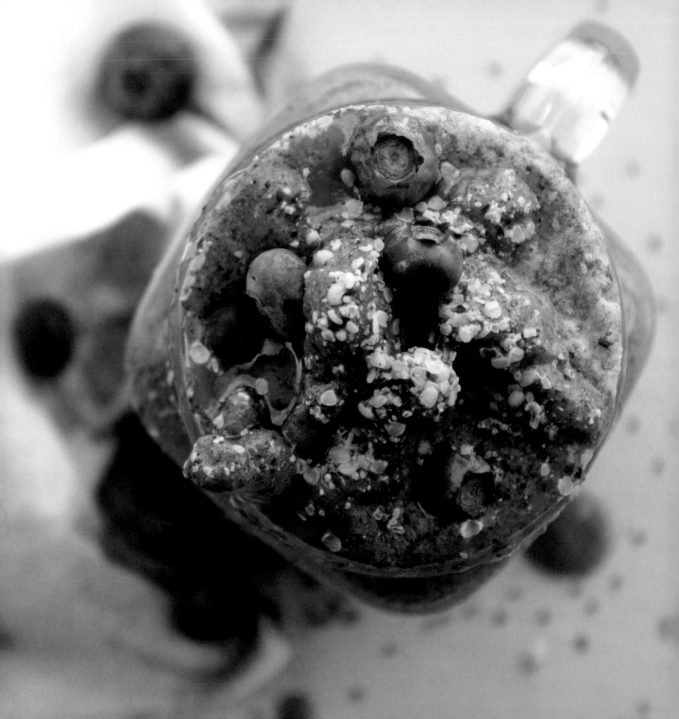

BLUE HIPPIE

Makes two 18-oz. servings

2 cups fresh or frozen organic blueberries

1 tbsp. chia seeds (powder)

1 tbsp. flaxseed (powder)

1 tbsp. hemp seed (powder)

1 tbsp. coconut oil

2 cups almond milk

Far out, man! Get the intense health boost of antioxidants in blueberries with the added benefits of hemp and flax seeds made creamy with almond milk. This drink will definitely make you one with the earthy flavors as well as help you feel totally groovy.

Place all ingredients into one blender and blend until smooth.

Personal Touch: _____

_____

_____

DAD'S FAVORITE

Juice: 36 oz.   Smoothie: three 12-oz. servings

½ head cabbage   8 oz. juice

3 stalks celery   1 banana

1 lb. carrots   1 large handful spinach

½ cucumber   1 large handful kale

½ apple   4–5 tbsp. blueberries

½ orange   2 tbsp. flaxseed

Juice.   Blend.

Dad's Favorite is as economically friendly as it is tasty. Juicing can be time consuming, but is a great way to capture high amounts of vitamins in one glass. To deliver a time-conscious, vitamin-packed punch and also get fiber in your daily diet, it's smart to combine the two. This recipe allows for two extra days of juice you can use for smoothie blending. Three days of vitamin-rich smoothies from one juicing session sounds like good economics to me.

Juice cabbage, celery, carrots, cucumber, apple, and orange. Pour juice into blender with all other ingredients and blend.

Personal Touch:

POST MARATHON

Makes two 18-oz. servings

1 banana

1 lemon

1 cup coconut water

1½ cups ice

1 cup water

One of the most integral parts to post-workout recovery is replacing lost fluids, and what better way to do that than with a superfood drink? Post Marathon's banana, citrus, and coconut combo meet these needs and are great for electrolyte replenishment. Starting a recovery routine is the best way to enhance overall workout performance and, with this drink, you are well on your way.

Blend all ingredients until smooth. Add protein or superfood powder, if necessary, and stir.

Personal Touch: _____

_____

_____

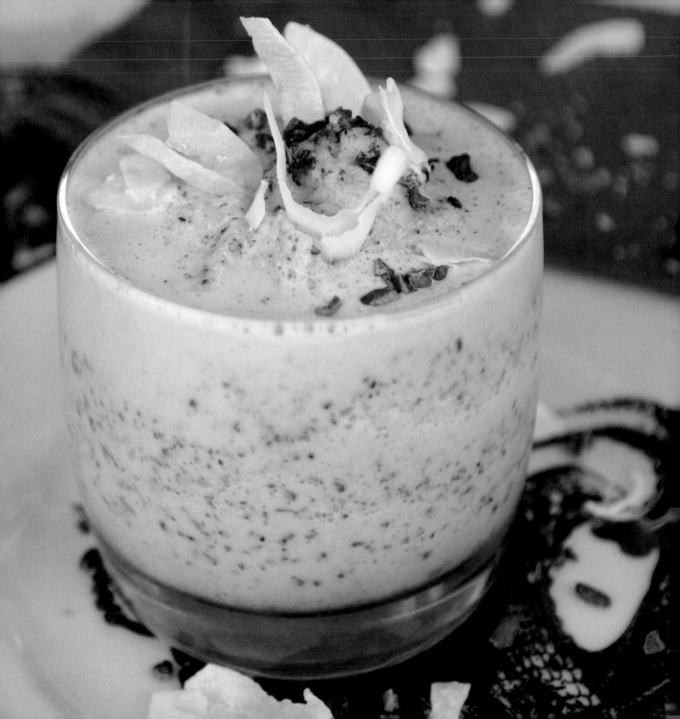

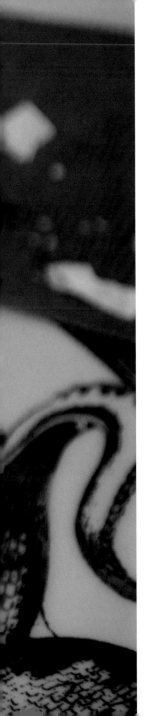

PALEO CHOCOLATE CHIP SMOOTHIE

Makes two 14-oz. servings

½ cup soaked almonds

½ coconut milk

½ cup coconut water

2 tbsp. cacao nibs

1 vanilla bean or 1 tsp. extract

1–2 tsp. pure maple syrup (optional)

½ tsp. sea salt

2 cups ice

You could say I have a bit of a cookie problem. It's sometimes difficult balancing good taste with a good diet. Our at-home Paleo Chocolate Cookie recipe inspired this next drink and had surprisingly positive results. Sweet and savory combinations, with the added plus of incorporating superfoods, gives you cookies-in-milk all at once without the unfortunate dilemma.

Skip the cookie sheet! Skin almonds and place in a blender with all other delicious ingredients. Blend until it resembles chocolate chip ice cream. Serve with a straw and enjoy the cacao crunch!

Personal Touch:

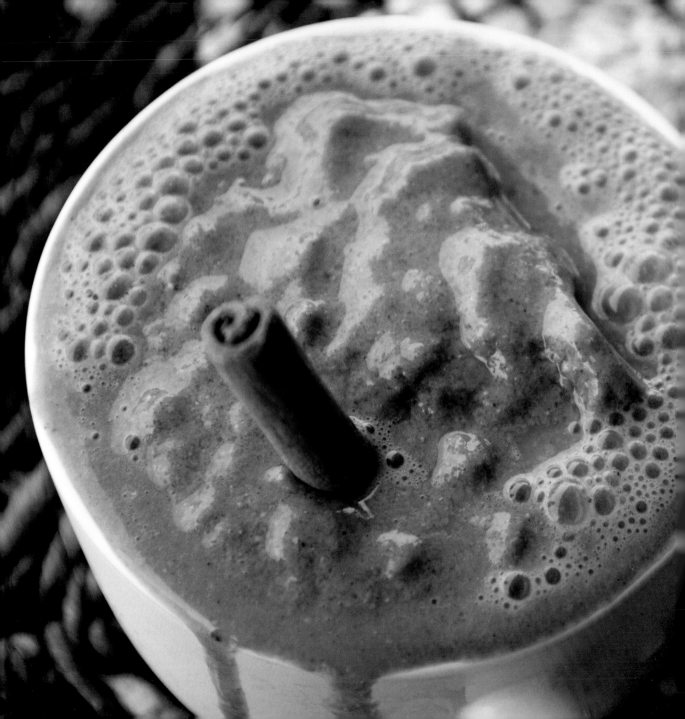

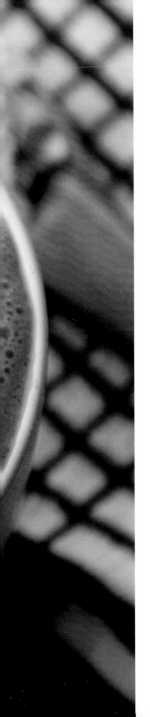

BREAKFAST SMOOTHIE

Makes two 18-oz. servings

1 frozen banana

½ cup organic rolled oats

2 tbsp. hemp seeds

1 tsp. maqui berry powder

1–2 cups water

1–2 cups ice

cinnamon and sea salt to taste

Quality time for breakfast most mornings is non-existent. This smoothie is something good you can do for yourself that won't take much time, but will send you out into the world fortified with a tasty drink that will stick to your ribs.

Blend all together in a high-powered blender. Dust with cinnamon and serve.

Personal Touch:

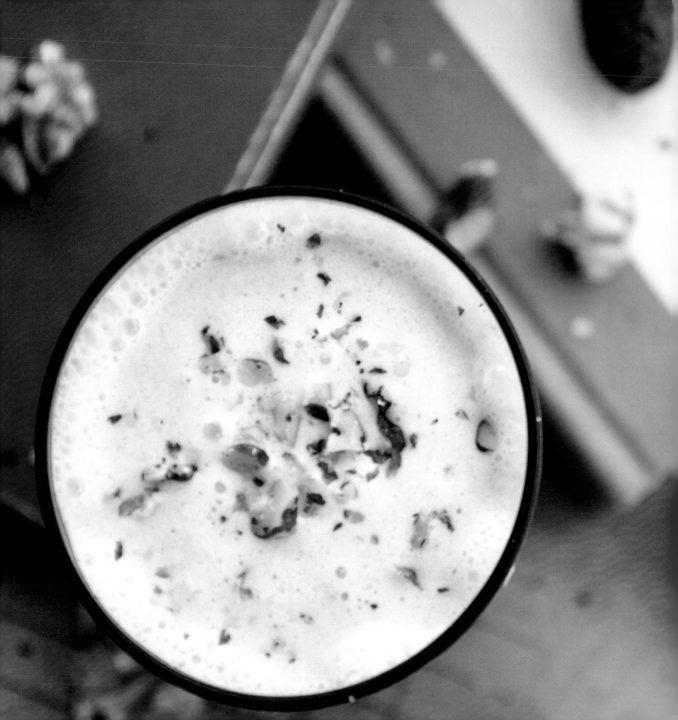

CREAMY WALNUT

Makes one 16-oz. serving

1 tbsp. flax seed

¼ cup soaked walnuts

2–3 dates (pitted)

½ cup organic whole milk yogurt

½ cup fresh young coconut water

1–2 cups ice

stevia to taste (optional)

The rich, natural flavor of walnuts combined with dates and yogurt bring out the nutty goodness of this drink. Flax seed delivers a fiber boost that is healthy and satisfying any time of the day.

Blend all ingredients together and enjoy!

Personal Touch:

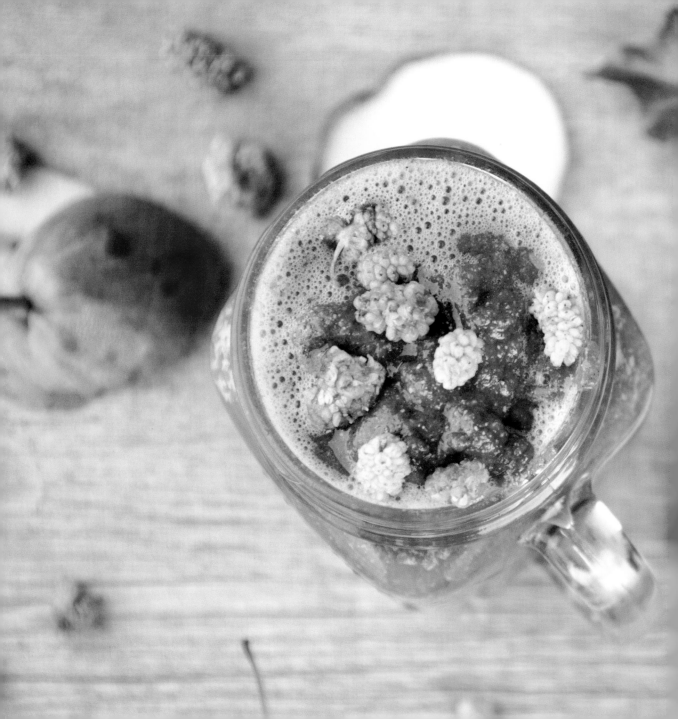

AUTUMN BOOST

Makes two 18-oz. servings

½ cup organic unsweetened pumpkin purée

½ overripe pear

2 tbsp. açaí powder

2 tbsp. flaxseed

2 tbsp. dried mulberries

1 cup coconut water

1 cup ice

Rich pumpkin promotes healthy skin, and high fiber combined with açaí age-defying benefits make this team a pretty tasty pair. This harvest time multi-superfood concoction is like pumpkin pie for your skin!

Blend all ingredients (except mulberries) together, sprinkle with mulberries, serve with a straw.

Personal Touch:

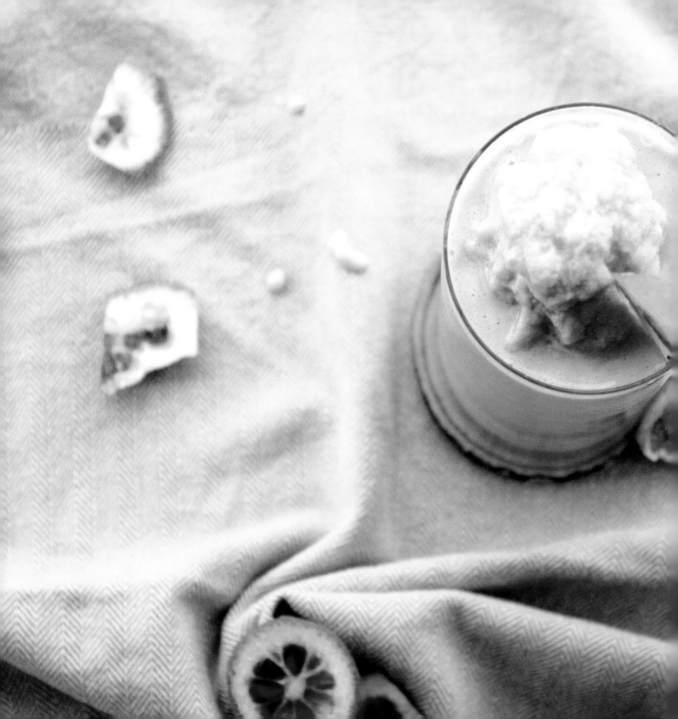

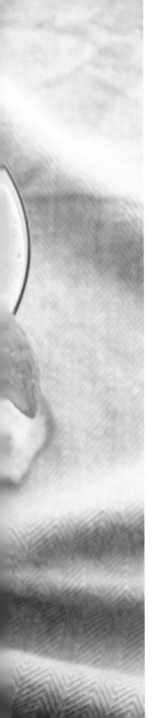

BLOOD ORANGE JULIUS

Makes two 18-oz. servings

1 blood orange (peeled)

1 cup organic whole milk yogurt

½ cup dried mulberries

1 vanilla bean or ½ tsp. extract

1 tsp. honey

½ cup coconut water

1½ cups ice

Pretty in pink, this creamy dreamsicle smoothie will absolutely surprise you. Its sinful flavor conceals its healthful nature. With every sip, you'd never guess you were taking in healthy probiotics, fighting disease, and reducing inflammation.

Juice blood orange and set aside. Blend all other ingredients together. Once blended, pulse blender to mix in the orange juice.

Personal Touch:

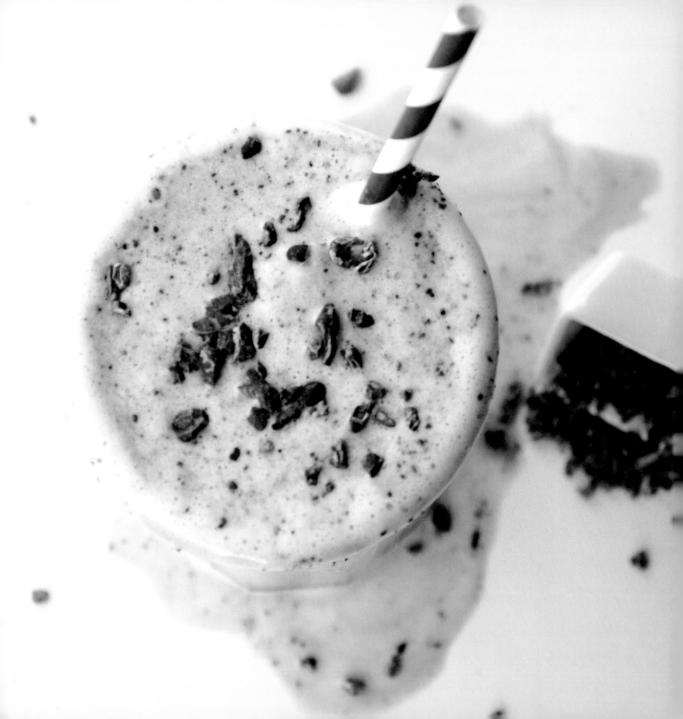

CHOCOLATE CHAI

Makes two 16-oz. servings

2 tbsp. flax seed

1 cup chai tea

½ cup organic raw whole milk

1 frozen banana

2 tbsp. cacao nibs

1 cup ice

Give in to the wonderful flavors of chocolate and banana melding together with a creamy chai tea. This combination is even more enjoyable when you know it is packing potassium and antioxidants in the same glass.

Blend all ingredients together in a high-powered blender.

Personal Touch:

BEAUTY BERRY

Makes one 12-oz. serving

1 ripe avocado

1 tbsp. soaked goji berries

1 tbsp. raw honey

½ cup whole milk yogurt

½ small cucumber juiced

1 cup coconut water

This drink couldn't be better for you if you wore it on your face. This one can make you beautiful on the inside as well as the outside.

Blend all ingredients together and serve with a straw.

Change it up: Reduce coconut water to ½ cup and blend to make a delectable face mask that combats dry skin. Apply with fingers, careful not to get too close to your eyes. This is a wet mask, so leave it on for about 25 minutes before rinsing off with warm water.

Personal Touch:

HEMP POWERED PROTEIN

Makes one 16-oz. serving

2 tbsp. hemp seed

1½ tbsp. cacao nibs

1½ cup frozen raspberries

½ cup whole milk yogurt

¼ tsp. turmeric

1 tbsp. chocolate protein powder

1 cup coconut water

Not your average protein drink, this sinful solution provides the tastiest recovery from a workout you've had that doesn't involve a cheat day. Fruity chocolate raspberry flavor blended with creamy coconut milk and yogurt with a savory hint of turmeric inspires you to skip that cheat day and keep reaching for your goal.

Place all ingredients in blender and blend until smooth.

Personal Touch:

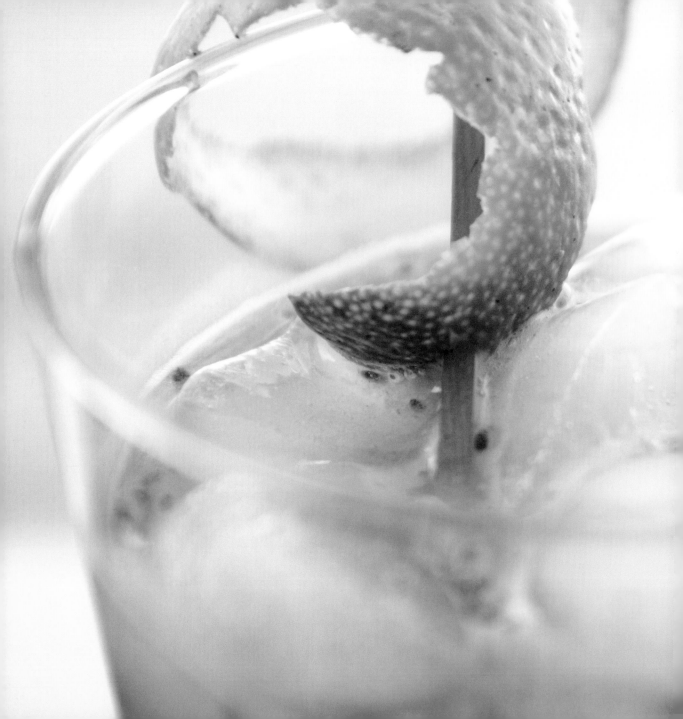

JUICES

Superfood juices require at the very least a juicer, but most incorporate superfood powders as well as infused ices, so a blender is highly recommended. By nature, these juices pack a very concentrated nutrient punch without the fiber to slow down absorption.

Components

FRUITS, SUPERFOODS, HERBS, SPICES, VEGETABLES

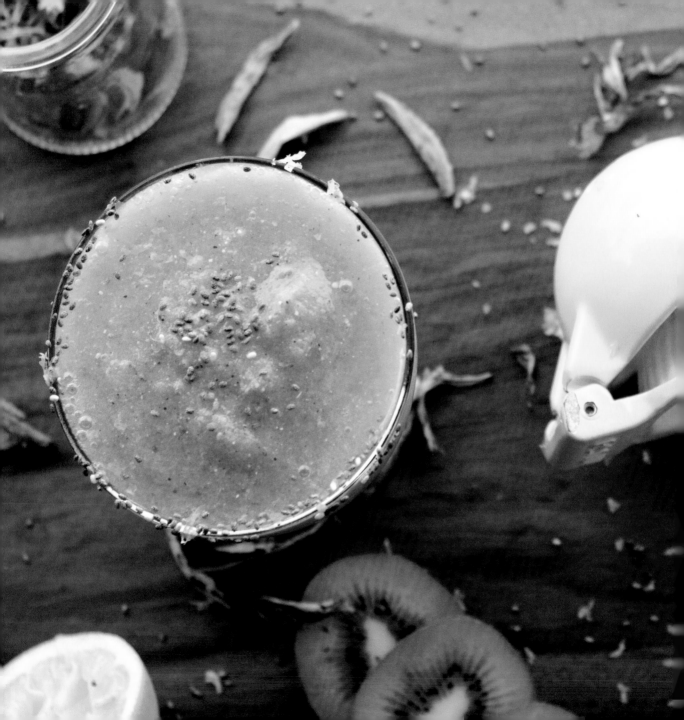

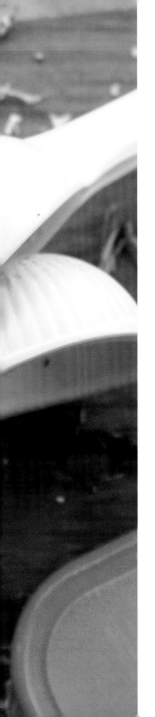

KIWI MELON
Makes one 16-oz. serving

1 kiwi (peeled)

½ lemon (peeled)

4 cups watermelon

chia seeds

Stevia to taste

Optional: add ice in blender

Kiwi and watermelon are a show-stopping flavor combination. The sweetness of the kiwi fruit paired with the brightness of the lemon and mellow melon flavors blend to make this drink a sure-to-be family juice favorite.

Personal Touch:

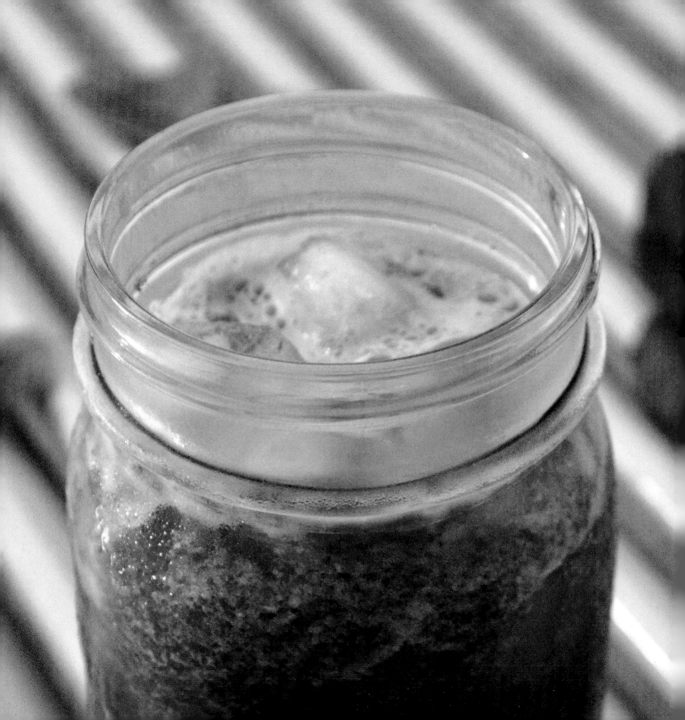

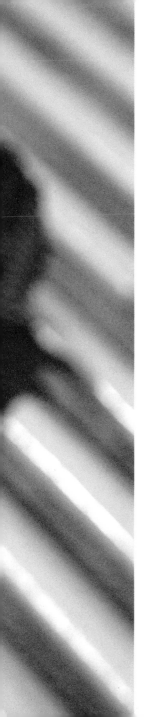

GREEN GLOW
Makes one 16-oz. serving

1 cup mint
2 cups spinach
3 cups pineapple
1 apple

Simple and delicious, Green Glow will have you glowing, too! This no-fuss recipe is a must for beginner juicers or young juice enthusiasts who aren't as seasoned with the experimental flavors of green drinks. I personally believe its easy prep and cleanup make it taste even better.

Juice all ingredients. Pour over ice and serve.

Personal Touch:

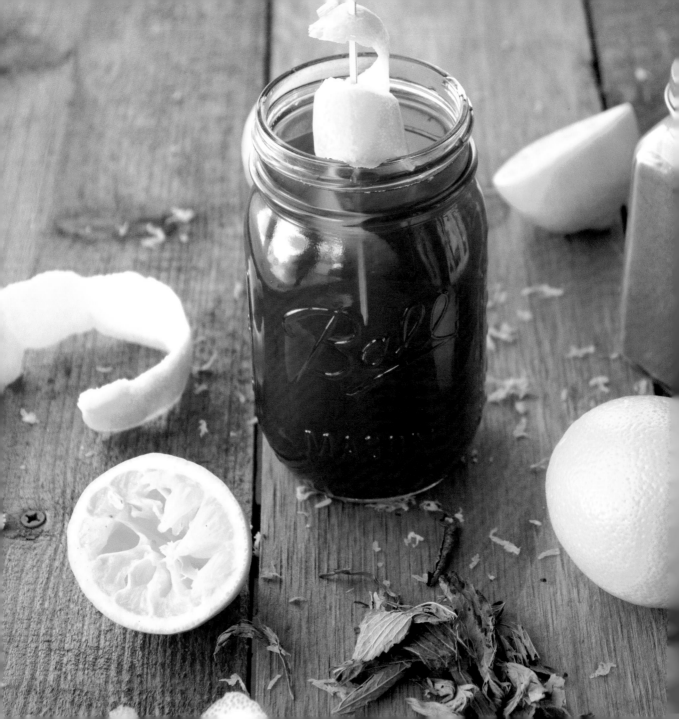

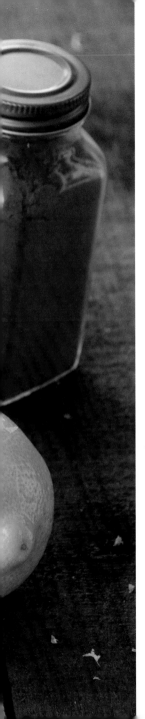

APPRENTICE CLEANSE

Makes two 16-oz. servings

2 lemons (peeled)

thumb of ginger

Stevia to taste

2 tsp. chlorella

¼ tsp. cayenne (optional)

2 cups water

If the Master had given his Apprentice a chance, he might have come up with this delicious elixir on his own. Chlorella adds so many additional benefits to this diet detox favorite, the very least of them being protein with little calorie increase. This wonderful blend of salty sweet flavors provides a gentle cleanse as a bonus.

Personal Touch:

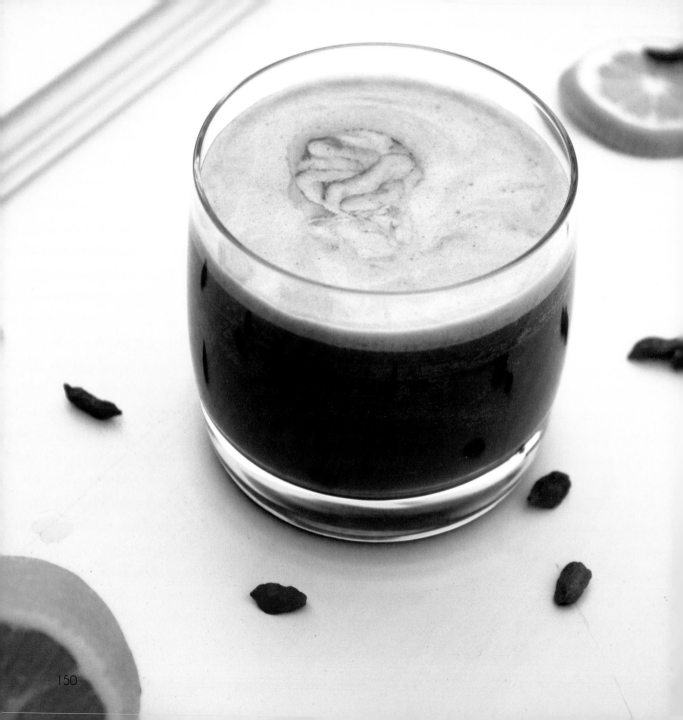

GOJI BEET

Makes one 16-oz. serving

1 small beet

1 orange

2 tbsp. soaked goji berries

2 lemons (peeled)

1 cup coconut water

Ancient Chinese knew the benefits of goji berries in mental wellbeing and calmness, athletic performance, happiness, and quality of sleep. In this recipe, they are all combined with coconut water, sour citrus, and earthy beet juice to make a delicious and healthful drink.

Juice orange, beet, and lemons. Pour juice in a blender with coconut water and goji berries and blend until smooth.

Personal Touch:

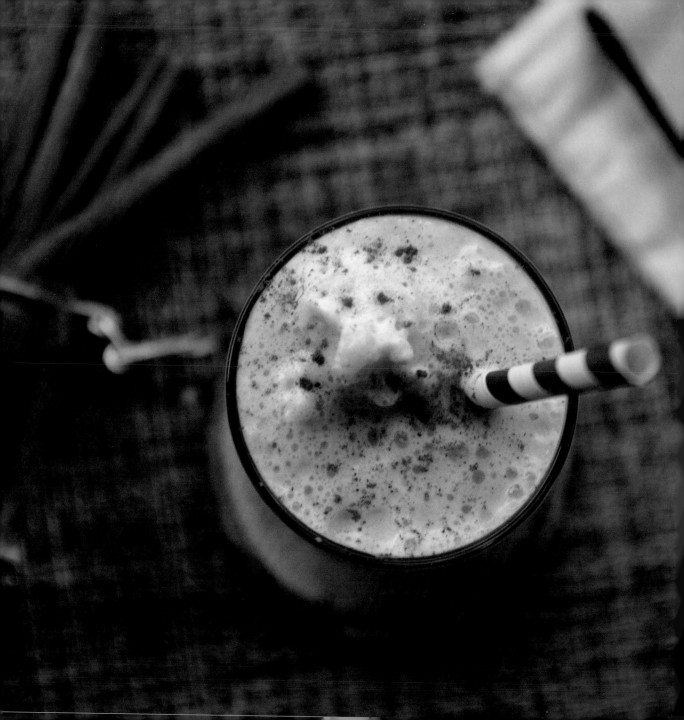

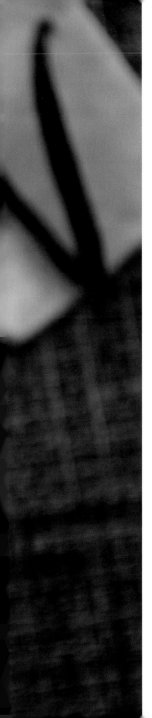

MACA MILK
Makes two 16-oz. servings

1 cup almond milk
1 tsp. maca powder (dependent)
¼ tsp. cinnamon
1 cup water
1 vanilla bean or 1 tsp. extract

Maca root is gaining popularity in the health community as being a superfood that delivers many positive benefits in just the smallest amount. Besides being beneficial to the circulatory system, it's also said to improve brain function and memory and reduce anxiety. This supplement should not be taken every day, and the dose should be gradually increased, starting at ½ teaspoon per serving.

Personal Touch: _____

_____

_____

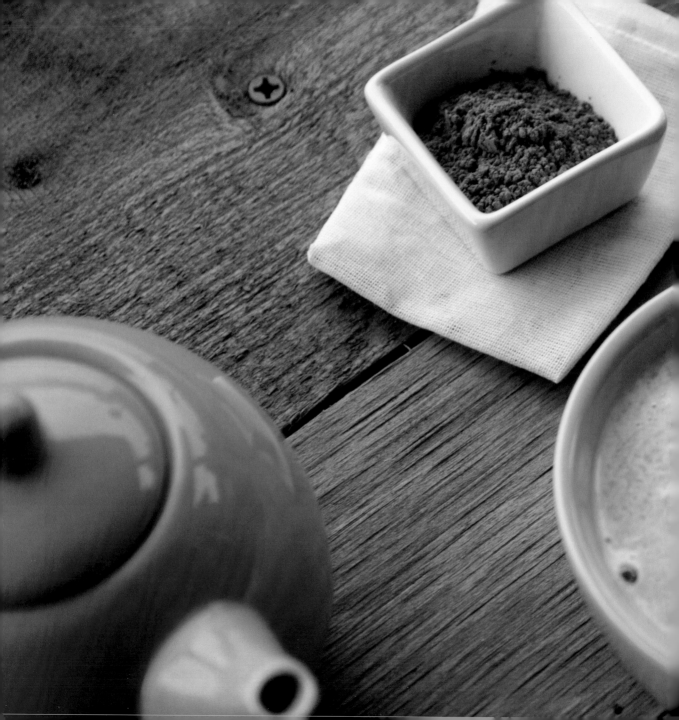

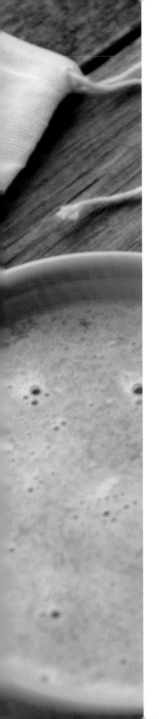

HONEY TEA

Makes one 16-oz. serving

1 cup green tea
2 cups honeydew melon
½ lemon

A healthy and great-tasting eastern world flavor, Honey Tea soothes you, mind, body, and soul. A nice way to end your daily yoga session, this drink will have you feeling as if are sitting full lotus on a bright spring day, refreshed among the cherry blossoms.

Make one cup of green tea. Stir in juiced honeydew with lemon. Serve warm.

Change it up:
Add mint and pour over ice for a relaxing eastern take on southern sweet tea.

Personal Touch:

CARRI-BEAN COOLER

Makes one 16-oz. serving

2 carrots

3 cups pineapple

3 bunches spinach

1 cup packed mint leaves

1 cup packed basil leaves

¼ jalapeño

2 tbsp. chia seeds

One glass of this and you'll think you've gone to heaven, if heaven were somewhere in the tropics where all the drinks are green and health is abundant. You wouldn't be entirely wrong. The sweet heat of this super juice will change the way you think of green drinks. Here's to the beginning of a healthier lifestyle.

Juice all fruits and vegetables. Pour over glass with ice and chia seeds, enjoy, and never go back. Bottoms up.

Personal Touch:

ORANGE LIQUORICE SODA

Makes one 16-oz. serving

3 blood oranges
2 kale leaves
1 small fennel bulb
1½ thumbs of ginger
1 cup mineral water

Our superfood Orange Liquorice Soda is an artisanal approach to superfood drinks. Spicy ginger, sweet blood oranges, and kale give you a fizzy lift while promoting heart health.

Juice oranges, ginger, kale, and fennel. Pour in a tall glass over ice. Stir in mineral water and enjoy.

Personal Touch:

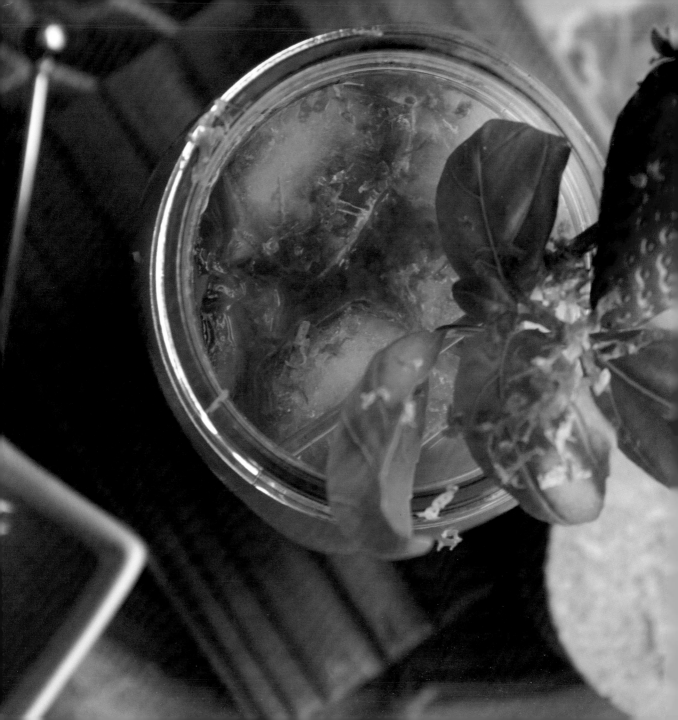

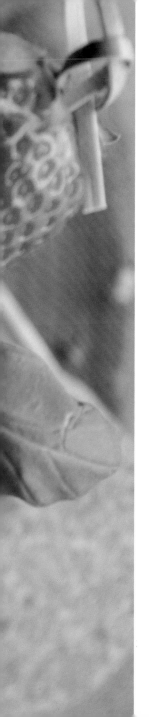

STRAWBERRY BASIL LIMEADE

Makes one 16-oz. serving

¼ cup packed basil leaves

2–3 leaves collard greens

5–6 strawberries

2 limes

1 cup mineral water

1–2 tbsp. honey (optional)

This is an all-time personal and crowd favorite. The flavor of strawberry provides a predictable sweetness, but is a great complement to the earthy green flavors of the collards and herbs. Lime punches up the sweetness of the strawberry, making this a delectable summer classic.

Juice all fruits and greens. Pour contents over ice and add mineral water.

Personal Touch:

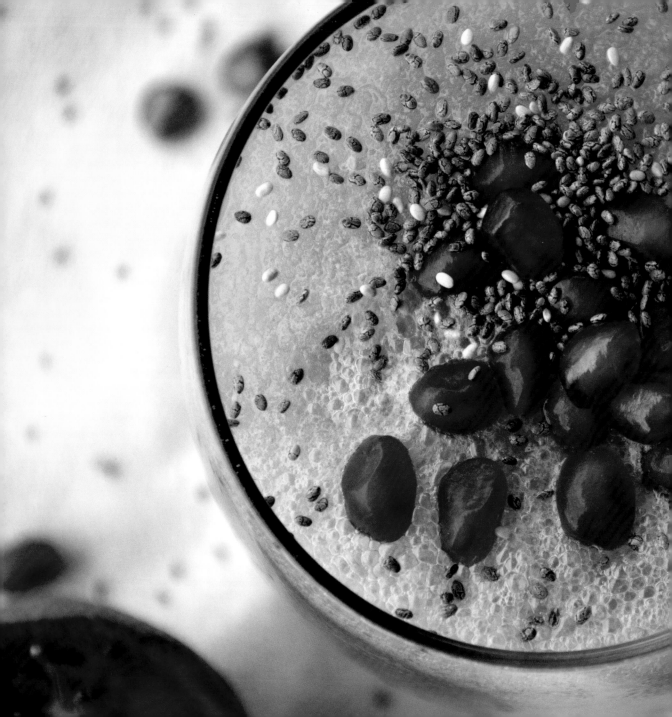

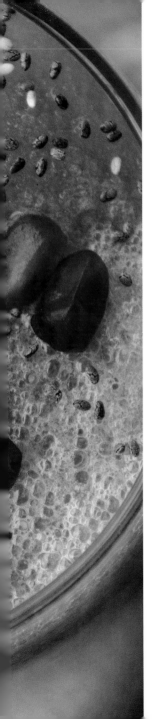

CAMU-DIG-IT?

Makes one 16-oz. serving

1 tsp. camu berry powder

½ cup pomegranate seeds

3 lemons

1 tsp. chia seeds

1 cup coconut water

1 cup ice

The key to any beauty regimen is water. So adding foods that promote hydration and cell replenishment is the best way to keep skin healthy and glowing. Chia seeds absorb water and increase the amount of water being delivered to the digestive tract, making it the perfect ingredient for this brilliant beauty cocktail.

Juice lemons. Add lemon juice to other ingredients in a blender and mix until pink.

Personal Touch:

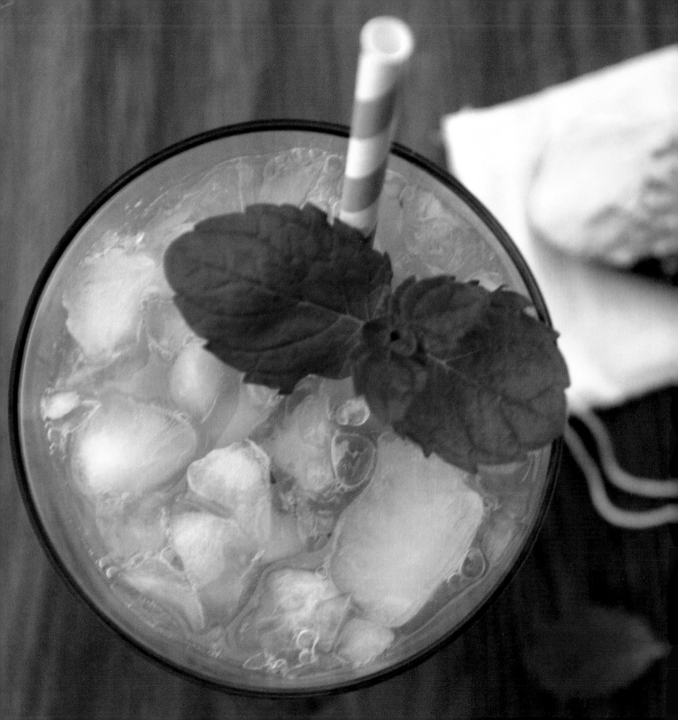

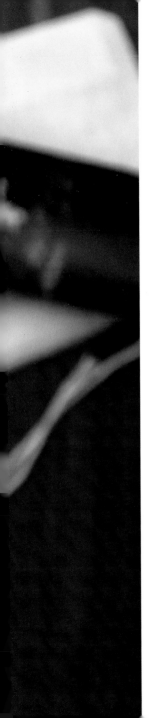

THE STRAW THAT BROKE THE CAMU'S BACK

Makes one 14-oz. serving

2 cups strawberry

1 tsp. camu powder

½ cup mint

1 cucumber

½ cup water

Camu camu berry is quickly becoming a popular health supplement due to its high antioxidant levels and antiviral properties. Being a native fruit of the Brazilian rainforest, it's not commonly found in your local grocer. However, you will most likely find it in powder form at a neighborhood health store. Adding it to any juice combination will only enhance its many health benefits.

Juice strawberries, cucumber, and mint. Pour juice mixture, water, and camu powder into blender and blend. Serve over ice or blend for a healthy camu slush.

Personal Touch:

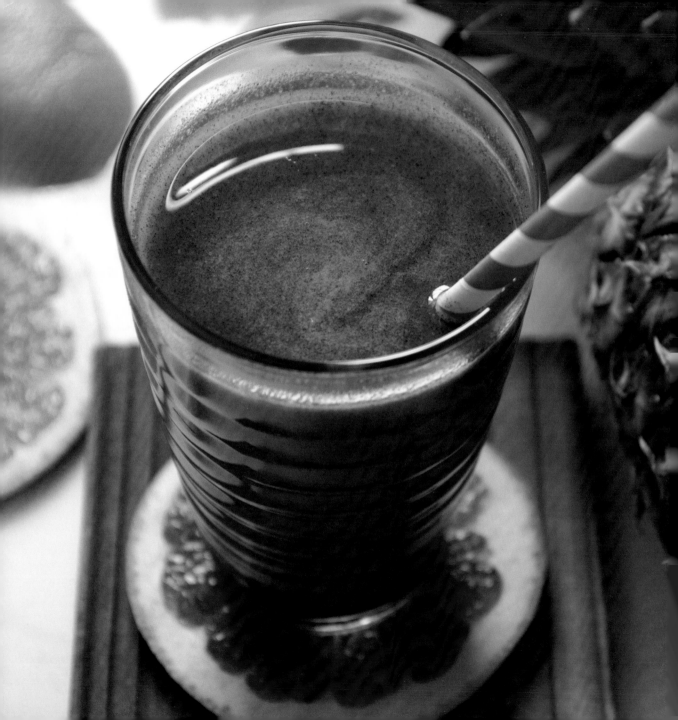

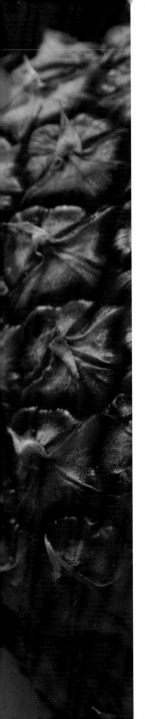

VITAMIN SEAWEED

Makes one 18-oz. serving

1 pink grapefruit (peeled)
2 cups pineapple
1 orange (peeled)
2 tsp. spirulina

Changing your diet isn't easy, and oftentimes it's hard to remember not to "drink your calories." Vitamin Seaweed makes this problem so much easier. A natural hunger-buster, pink grapefruit is also said to help boost your metabolism. Getting the proper amount of protein is also important with any diet, and spirulina is a great source of protein and nutrients. This drink is also really great for vegetarians and pregnant mothers looking to add protein to their diets.

Juice fruit and pour over ice into glass with spirulina. Cover, shake, and serve.

Personal Touch:

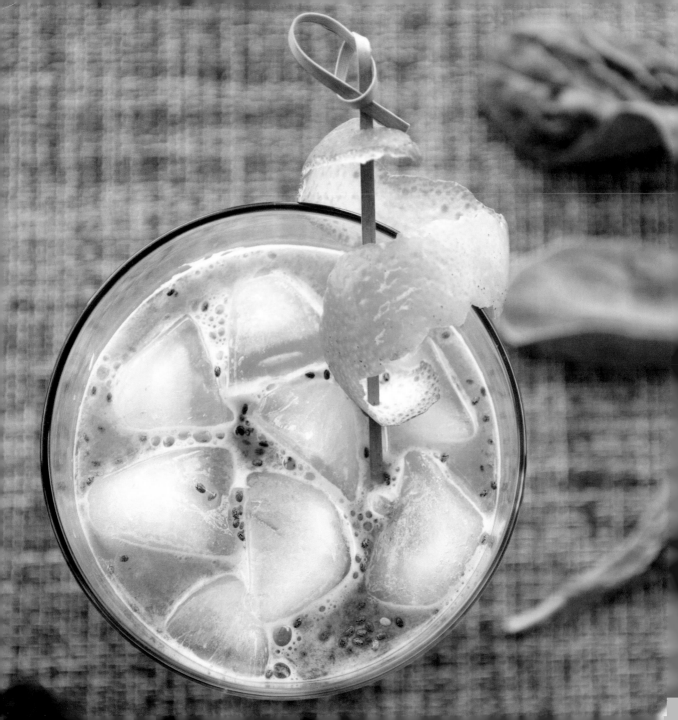

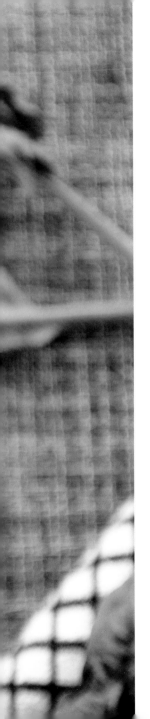

COOLAIDE

Makes one 16-oz. serving

2 cups spinach

½ cup mint

2 limes (peeled)

thumb of ginger

1–2 tsp. chia seeds

1 cup water

Green means go! Kids and kids at heart will love this neon green tangy summer limeade. It looks nearly as electric as it makes you feel. Great for a backyard barbeque or at the pool where playing all day can really take it out of you.

Juice all greens, fruit, and ginger. Pour over ice and chia seeds. Stir with a spoon and serve.

Personal Touch:

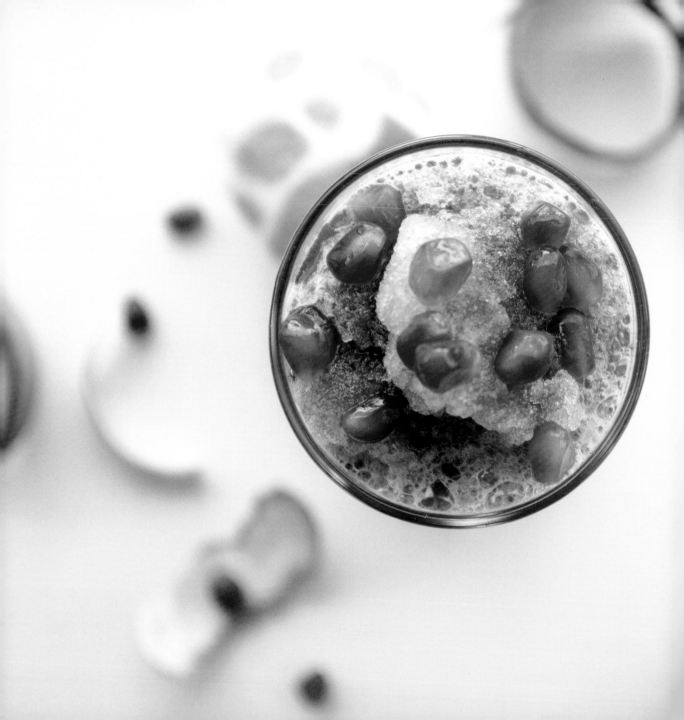

CUTECUMBER

Makes one 14-oz. serving

2 cucumbers
½ cup basil
1 lime (peeled)
½ pomegranate seeds
1 tsp. chlorella

Feel like you could use a day at the spa, but you don't have the time? If you've got a juicer, these ingredients, and a few minutes, you may not have that Swedish massage, but you're one step closer to feeling much better. Chlorella contains high detox properties to help rid your body of nasty toxins and, to top it off, is said to slow the aging process. Toss in the high antioxidants that fight cell-damaging free radicals, and you've got yourself one tasty anti-aging cocktail.

Juice all solid ingredients. Pour juice into glass over chlorella, stir to mix, and add ice. Save two cucumber slices to rest on your eyelids as you enjoy this beauty beverage.

Personal Touch:

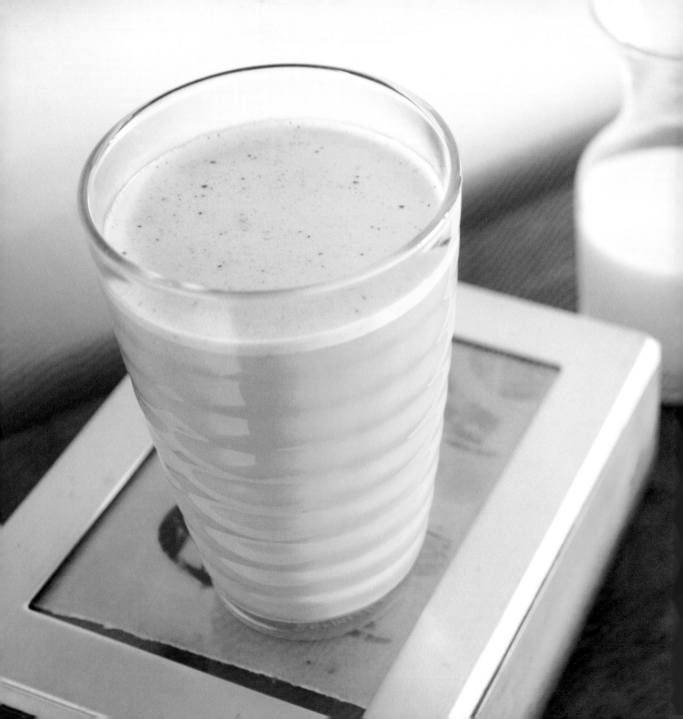

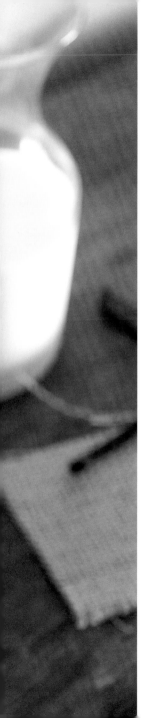

CARROT SPICE
Makes two 16-oz. servings

1 cup carrot juice
¼ cup fennel juice
¾ cup organic raw whole milk
¼ tsp nutmeg
1 vanilla bean or ½ tsp. extract

If you are having a hard time choosing between your orange juices in the morning, let us help you make it easier. Carrot Spice takes a sophisticated stand as "the other" morning orange juice drink. Just like oranges, carrots contain high levels of vitamin C, but have many other properties attributed to cancer fighting and detoxing.

Adding grass-fed whole milk and fennel not only adds digestive health and reducing inflammation to the list of benefits, but creates an earthy and creamy sweetness that makes it an easy choice for your go-to "orange" juice.

Juice carrots and fennel. Add all ingredients and juice to the blender and blend until milky.

Personal Touch:

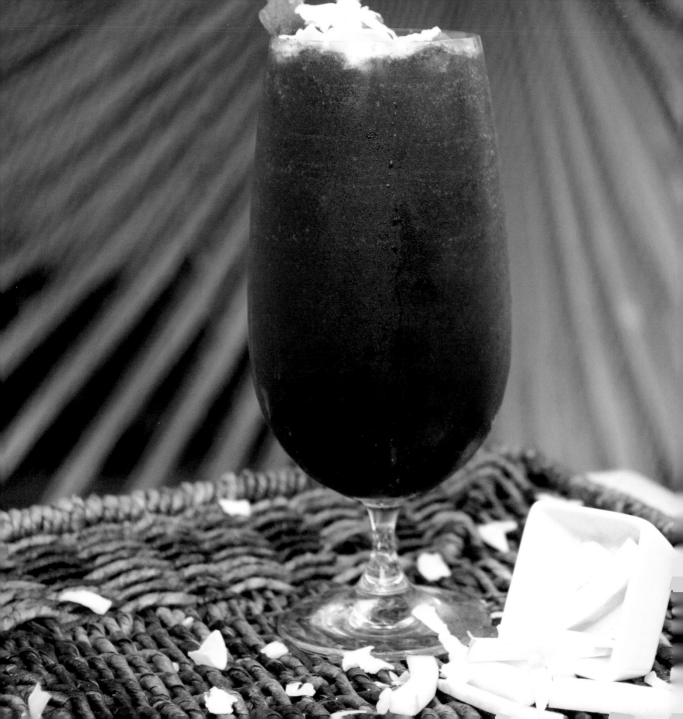

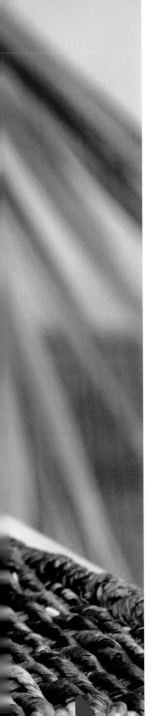

BEACH PEACH

Makes one 14-oz. serving

2 peaches (pitted)
1 thumb ginger
1 tsp. açaí powder
1 tsp. spirulina
½ cup fresh young coconut water
shake with ice

Helping your body to detox never tasted so good. Spirulina is known to bind with toxins and heavy metals in your bloodstream and help remove them. Another way to cleanse your body is to ensure you have enough dietary fiber. Açaí berries are a high-fiber fruit that have powerful detoxification capacities. Healthy cell regeneration is key for any detox, and the high electrolyte count of coconut water helps to hydrate and replenish cells. All these components together make for a powerful and delicious detox treat.

Juice peaches and ginger. Pour into a glass with açaí powder and spirulina and stir. Shake with ice and serve.

Personal Touch:

INFUSED WATERS

Too many of us avoid water because, let's face it, it's pretty boring and lacks the flavor our generation insists be present. No need to reach for the many varieties of bottled flavored water on the shelf, most with unhealthy added sugars, when we can quickly and easily make our own right at home.

Water helps control calories, aids with digestion, absorbs nutrients, improves circulation of blood, encourages creation of saliva, maintains body temperature, and helps flush the body of toxins. We are 60 percent water; it is essential to life itself, so let's make it easier to consume.

Pick and choose from one or more of the following five components of infused waters: fruits (berries, apple, kiwi, etc.), vegetables (carrots, celery, etc.), herbs (basil, mint, rosemary, etc.), spices (pepper, cinnamon, etc.), and waters (tap, filtered, mineral, etc.).

5 Components of Infused Waters

FRUITS, VEGETABLES, HERBS, SPICES, WATERS

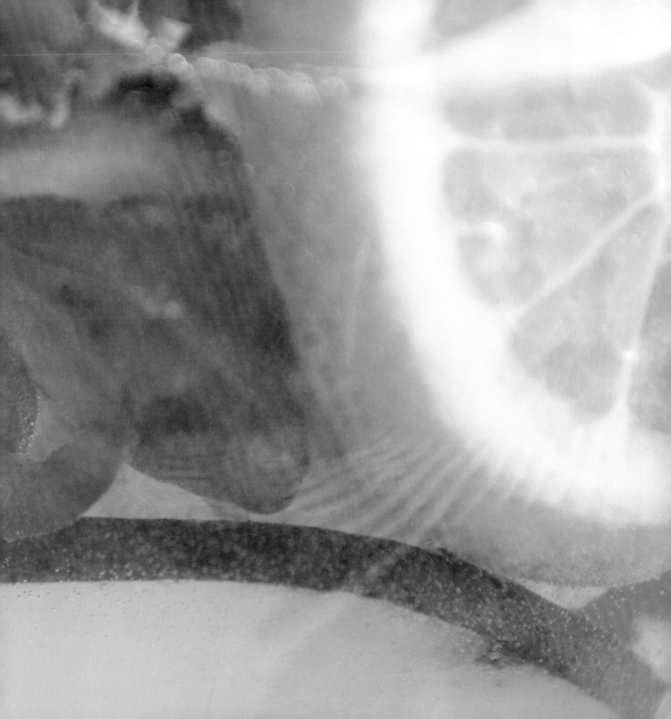

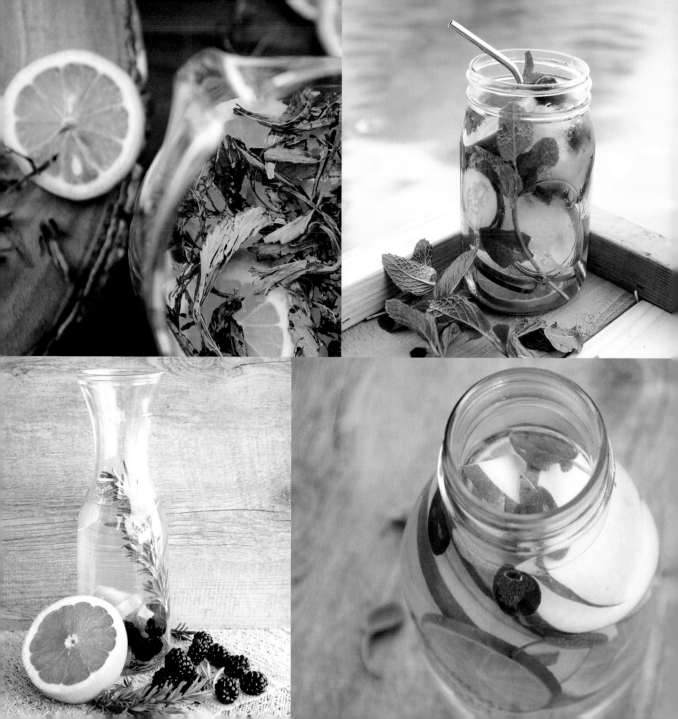

SWEET & SPICY CITRUS

8 cups water
1 tangerine, thinly sliced
1 Meyer lemon, thinly sliced
1 pear, thinly sliced
1 red Thai chili pepper, thinly sliced
4–5 sprigs cilantro

SAGE, APPLE, LIME

8 cups water
1 apple, thinly sliced
1 lime, thinly sliced
2–3 leaves sage

BLACKBERRY, GRAPEFRUIT, ROSEMARY

8 cups water
6–8 blackberries
½ grapefruit, thinly sliced
1 sprig rosemary

WATERMELON MINT

8 cups mineral water
2 cups watermelon, cubed
2–3 sprigs mint

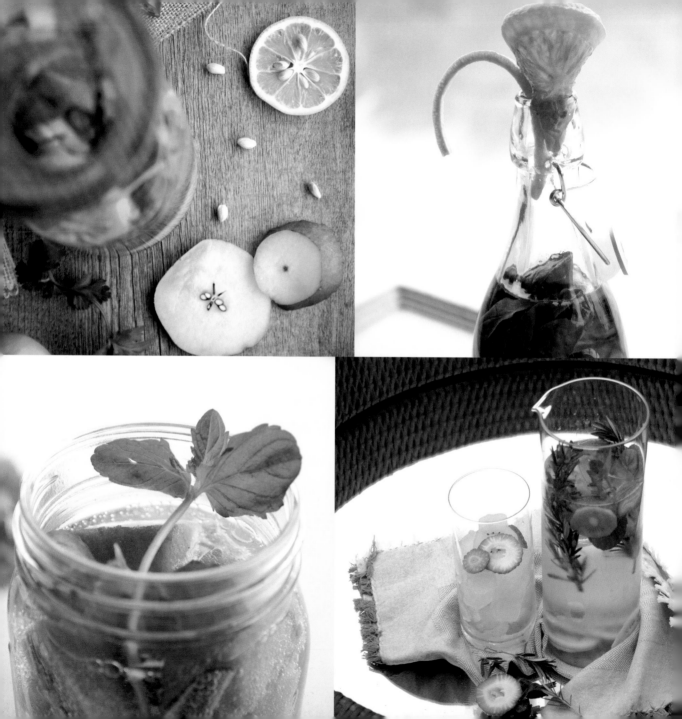

CUCUMBER CHERRY MINT

8 cups water
1 small cucumber, thinly sliced
1 lime, thinly sliced
6-8 cherries, pitted
2-3 sprigs mint

PINEAPPLE LEMON

8 cups water
2 cups pineapple, cubed
1 lemon, thinly sliced
4-6 leaves Stevia

STRAWBERRY KIWI ROSE-MINT

8 cups mineral water
2-3 strawberries, thinly sliced
1 kiwi, thinly sliced
2-3 sprigs mint
1 sprig rosemary

BLOOD ORANGE BASIL

8 cups mineral water
1 blood orange, thinly sliced
2-3 leaves basil

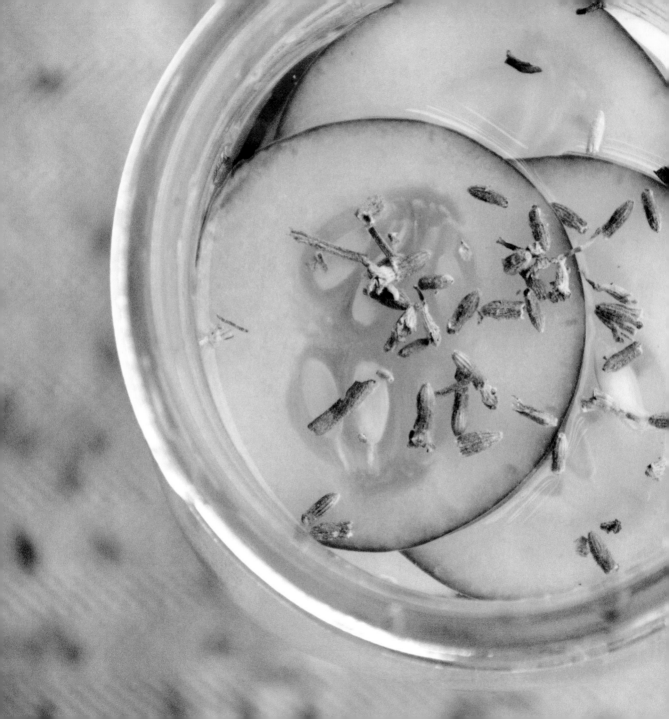

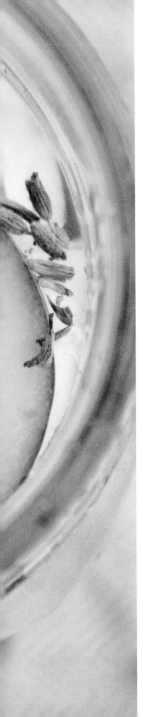

CUCUMBER LAVENDER

8 cups water

1 tsp. dried lavender

1 small cucumber, thinly sliced

This delicate drink is a powerful example of the benefits and ease of infused waters. Bright perfumes of herbs like lavender are muted and tamed by the presence of other fruits and vegetables, like cucumber, in water, allowing you to fully receive all the positives of the ingredients without overwhelming your palette with aromatics and flavors that may be semi-volatile.

Personal Touch:

COFFEE, TEA & OTHER DRINKS

Served hot or over ice, combining superfoods with most teas adds flavor as well as a higher nutrient value to an everyday beverage.

Components

FRUITS, SUPERFOODS, HERBS, SPICES, TEAS

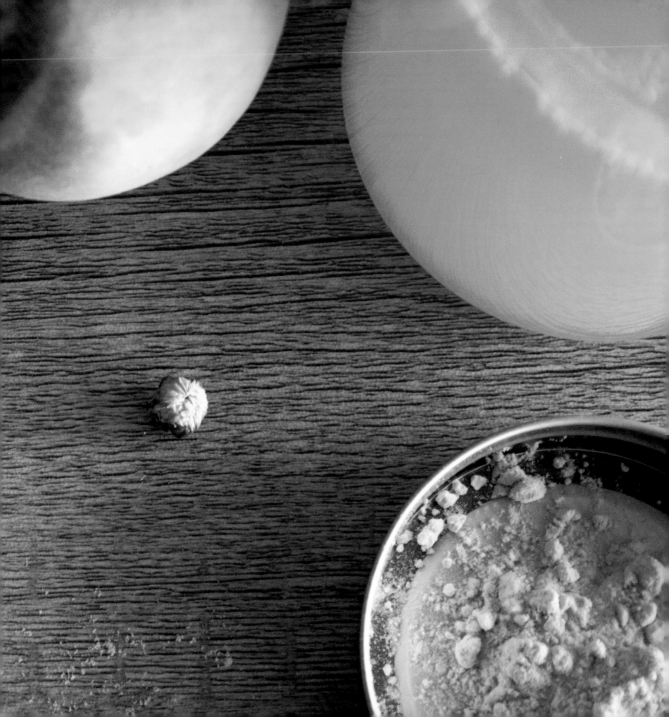

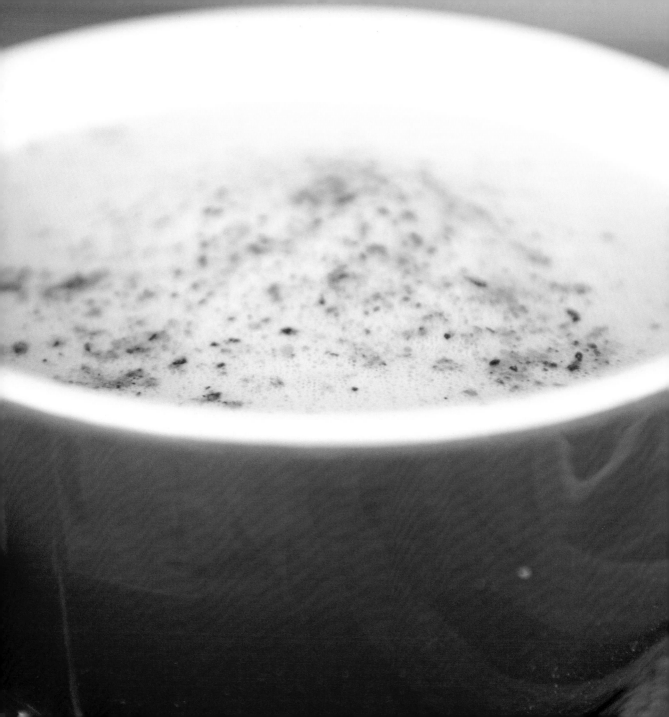

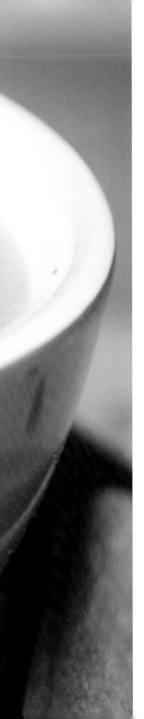

EGGS & COFFEE

Makes one 10-oz. serving

1 cup coffee

2–3 raw organic pastured egg yolks

½ tsp. cinnamon

1 tsp. turmeric

pinch of salt

honey or stevia to sweeten

Is coffee really good for you? It leads to better blood circulation, it boosts the metabolism, and thus supports a healthy heart. What you put inside your coffee really makes all the difference. Eggs & Coffee has just the thing to get your morning routine started right. Organic pastured egg yolks add a creamy texture, making this a perfect on-the-go breakfast drink. Cinnamon is a great substitute for sugar, as it is far healthier, adds flavor, and helps regulate blood sugar. So I ask again, is coffee really good for you? What do you think?

Brew up one cup of coffee. Toss fresh coffee into blender with all remaining ingredients. Blend until creamy. Serve in your favorite coffee carry-out cup.

Personal Touch:

185

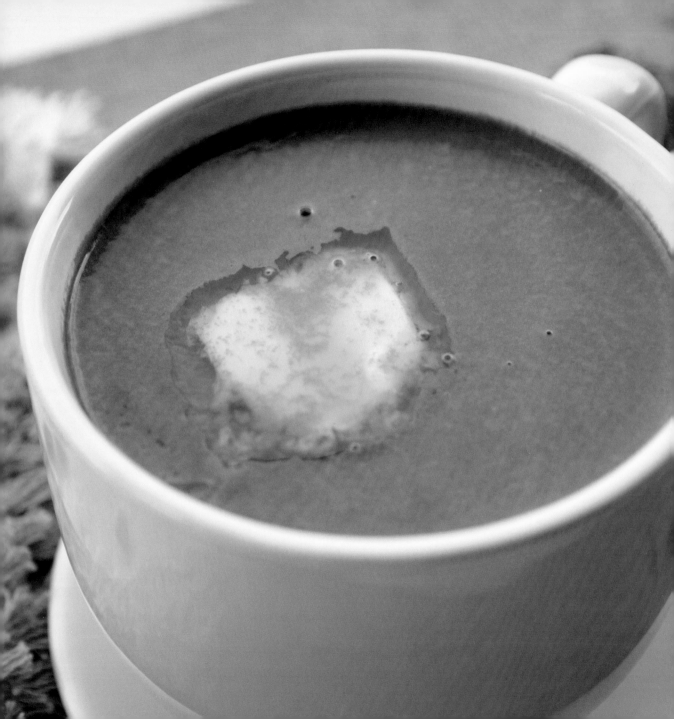

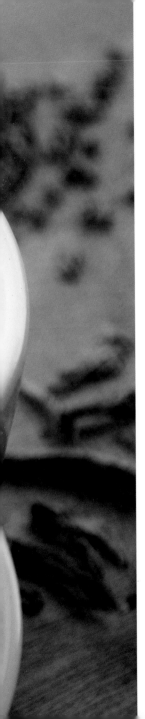

COCOBUTTER BREW

Makes one 9-oz. serving

1 cup coffee

1 tsp. cacao powder

1–2 tbsp. organic grass-fed butter (unsalted)

1 tbsp. organic virgin coconut oil

Stevia to sweeten

This is a popular coffee drink among the paleo community. As the paleo lifestyle supports the concept of healthy proteins and the lack of refined sugars or grains, it leaves many paleo enthusiasts saying, "So what can I put in my coffee?" CocoButter Brew is a superfood solution to ensure a healthier way to wake up.

Brew 1 cup of your favorite coffee. Pour into blender with all other ingredients. Blend until smooth.

Personal Touch:

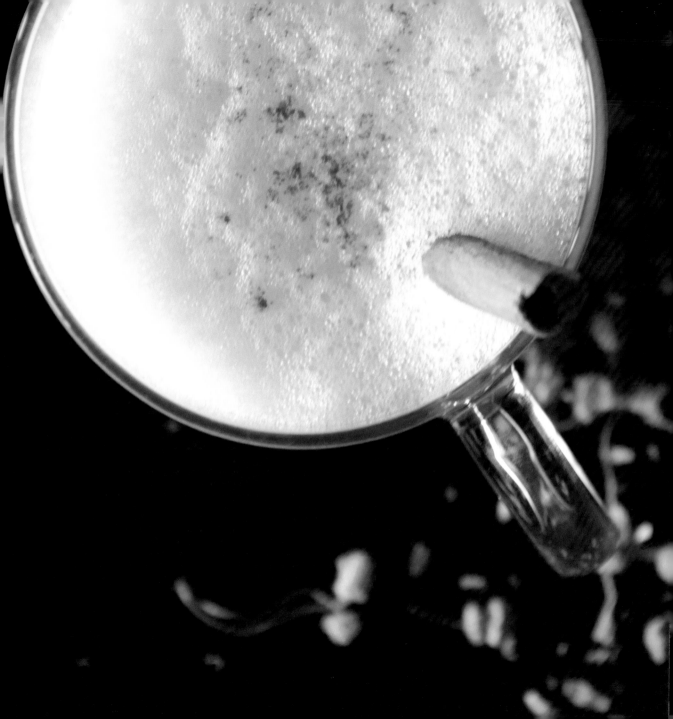

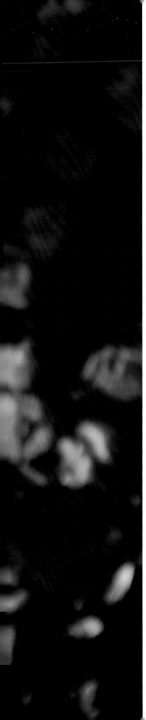

CHAMOMILK

Makes one 10-oz. serving

1 cup chamomile tea

¼ cup organic raw whole milk

1–2 raw organic pastured egg yolks

honey or stevia to sweeten

Stress can be a killer, and we all need a way to unwind. So much of what we put in our bodies every day can help support or reduce stress. Most of our daily diets are high in omega-6 acids, which are attributed to inflammation in the brain and have been linked to mood fluctuation. Increasing your intake of omega-3 fatty acids is a great way to start to treat stress. Adding healthy whole milk from grass-fed cows and pastured egg yolks to a tried and true stress reliever like chamomile tea is a recipe for relaxation.

Personal Touch:

BUTTERSCOTCH ICED CHAI LATTE

Makes one 12-oz. serving

1 cup chai tea

1 tsp. maca powder

2 tbsp. whole milk

1 thumb of ginger

¼ tsp. cinnamon

Stevia if necessary

1½ cup ice

Buttery maca root enhances the bold, warm flavors of old-world chai tea to create a smooth spiced way to give you a boost of energy to start off the day or a workout. Not meant for everyday use, maca is said to help enhance athletic performance and improve stamina. Maca also has properties to support beauty, as it is known to help restore red blood cells and reduce acne. The anti-inflammatory effects of ginger also make this a great recipe for overall beauty health and a creamy complement to a long hike or day at the gym.

In a blender, combine cooled chai tea with all other ingredients. Blend until smooth and creamy. Pour into your favorite on-the-go cold drink container and take on the day.

Personal Touch:

LAVENDER ZINGER

Makes two 8-oz. servings (2 quarts lavender/mint water)

1 tsp. loose leaf lavender

1 tsp. camu powder

4 medium mint leaves

Fresh mint and camu berries add a sour tang to the clean taste of lavender tea to make this drink taste something reminiscent of the traditional Lemon Zinger. Although it lacks the lemon component, it packs thirty times the vitamin C punch of any lemon, thanks to the camu powder. Lavender's antiseptic properties are often used to treat digestive issues and has been said to help combat insomnia and anxiety. This tea is great for study sessions during cold season.

Add 2 quarts of water to lavender and mint leaves to a saucepan or tea kettle and bring all to a boil. Reduce heat and simmer for 10 minutes. Strain 2 cups into blender with camu powder. Blend and serve. Also great over ice.

Personal Touch:

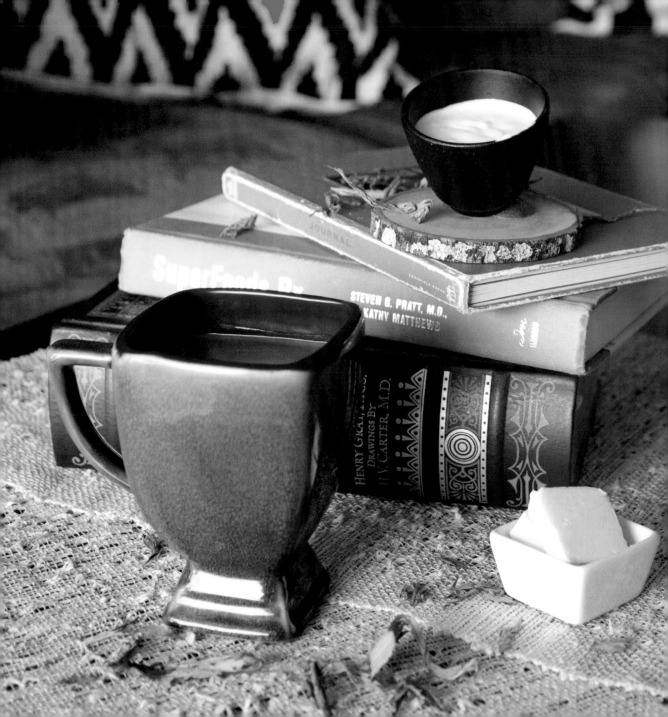

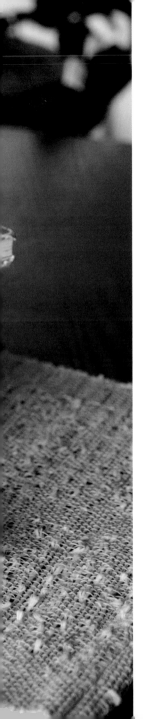

FROTHY CHAI LATTE

Makes one 10-oz. serving

1 cup chai tea
1 organic raw pastured egg
1 tbsp. organic coconut milk
1–2 tbsp. organic grass-fed butter (unsalted)
¼ tsp. vanilla extract
Stevia to sweeten

The double energy boost you get from Frothy Chai Latte is a great way to start any day or recharge on a cool afternoon. Besides the caffeine boost, grass-fed butter adds not only great flavor, but gives you lots of energy and healthy fats that your body will use to make cell walls and hormones.

Combine hot chai and all ingredients in blender and blend until frothy.

Change it up:
If you're looking to avoid caffeine, a few household spices you may find in your kitchen are good substitutes.
2 cinnamon sticks
6 cardamom pods
10 whole cloves
2 tsp. black peppercorns
1 date, pitted for sweetness

Combine lightly bruised spices in a teapot with 2 quarts of water. Bring to a boil, then reduce to a simmer for 10 minutes. Strain contents into blender. Add date, egg, butter, coconut milk, and vanilla. Blend until frothy, then pour warm contents into mug. Heat to taste. Dust with ground cinnamon and serve.

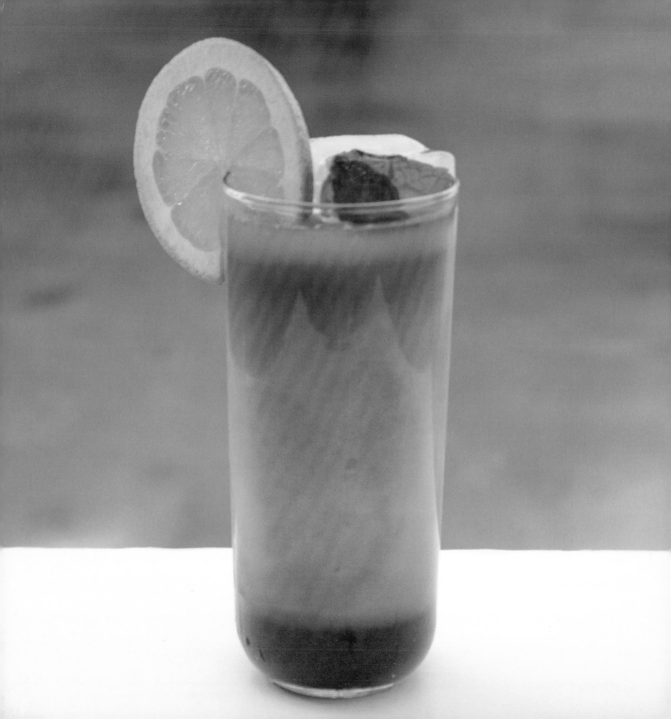

LA GREEN TEA

Makes one 12-oz. serving

½ cup green tea (chilled)
½ cup orange juice
½ cup pomegranate juice
squirt of lemon

This is a spa day antioxidant powerhouse in a glass. Green tea, pomegranate, and lemon work together to fight cell degeneration, slow the aging process, and promote healthy vibrant skin. Feeling so good on the inside never looked so good on the outside.

Juice pomegranate separately, juice the orange and lemon together, and mix tea and water in a separate glass. In a tall glass over ice, pour in pomegranate juice first, followed by the orange juice very slowly, and finally, the green tea.

Personal Touch:

GINGER FENNEL TEA

Makes two 8-oz. servings (2 quarts fennel/ginger/orange water)

1–2 tsp. crushed fennel seeds
1 thumb of ginger
juice of ½ an orange
dried peel of 1 orange (optional)

Smooth and zesty, this tea packs a superfood one-two punch for common stomach issues. Ginger, being an anti-inflammatory, naturally battles nausea or cramping, while fennel is a known diuretic that helps with constipation. The oil and fiber from orange peels combats indigestion and soothes the digestive system.

Battling a long day or fighting an upset stomach just got a little easier.

Fill a teapot with 2 quarts of water. Add fennel, ginger, and peel. Bring water to a boil, then reduce heat and simmer for 10 minutes. Pour two cups of tea through a strainer into your favorite mug, stir in orange juice, and serve.

Personal Touch: _____

_____

_____

SUPER ICED MOCHA

Makes two 16-oz. servings

1 cup coffee

½ cup coconut milk

1 tbsp. raw cacao nibs

2 tbsp. hemp protein powder

1 tsp. cinnamon

½ tsp. nutmeg

1 tsp. honey

1½ cups ice

You don't need to hit the neighborhood coffee shop for the taste of a designer mocha that cools you down on a hot day. Cut the trip and the calories by blending one up at home using multiple superfoods.

Brew up a cup of your favorite coffee. Combine coffee, coconut milk, cacao nibs, honey, cinnamon, and nutmeg in a blender over ice and blend until smooth. Serve up in a tall glass, sprinkle with crushed cacao nibs, and drink with a straw.

Personal Touch:

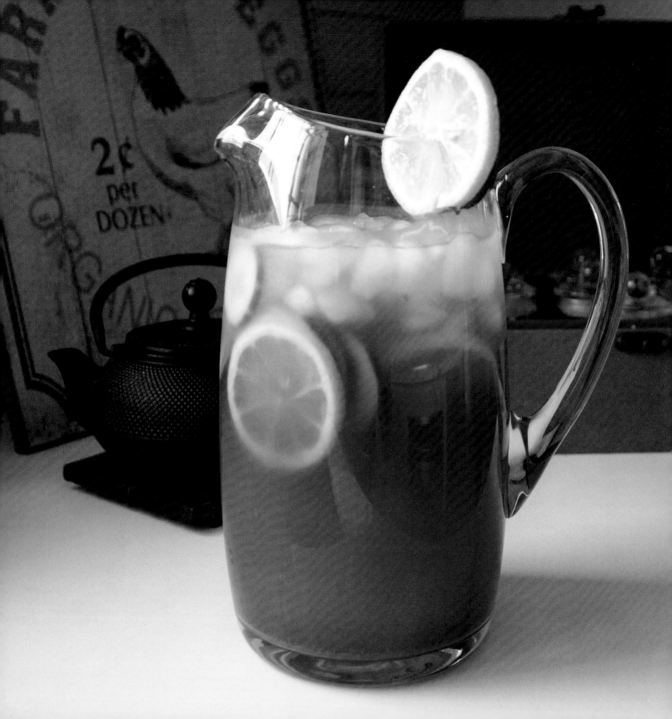

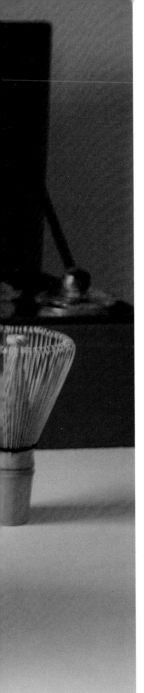

CUCUMBER TEA
Makes two 18-oz. servings

1 tsp. matcha tea
3–4 slices cucumber
2 slices lemon
2 cups water (warm)
ice

Hydration is the most important part of cleanses; in general, hydration helps you live cleaner day to day. What you use to ensure regular fluid replenishment will absolutely make a difference in your detox. Matcha green tea as a natural laxative helps to push toxins out of your system. Cucumbers, being 95 percent water, are optimal for fluid replenishment.

Brew matcha tea. Add ice. Pour in juiced cucumbers and lemon and stir.

Personal Touch:

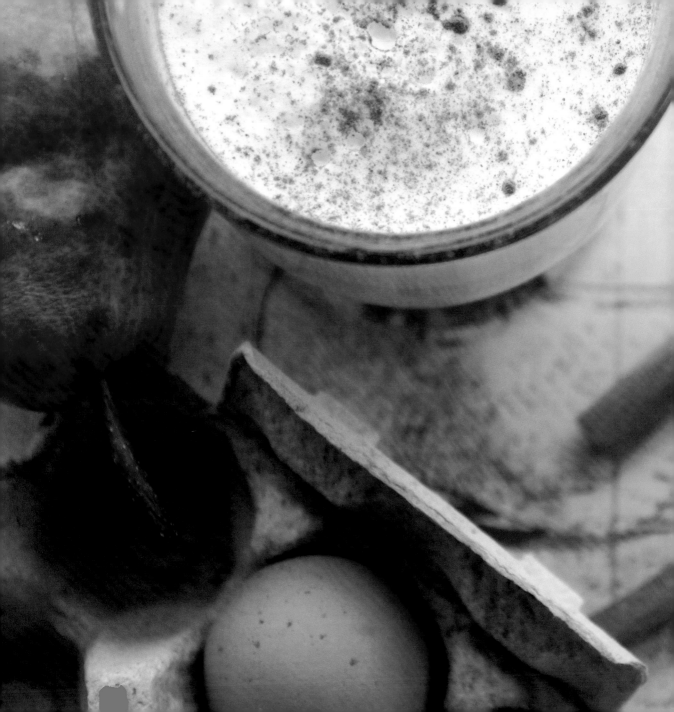

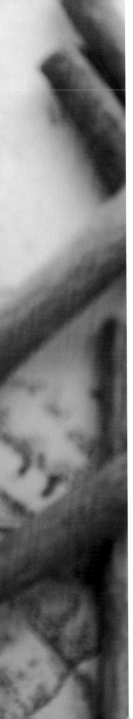

PEAR APPLE CIDER

Makes one 8-oz. serving

1 Anjou pear (juiced)
2 red apples (juiced)
thumb of ginger (juiced)
4 cinnamon sticks
1 organic pastured egg white

Mulled spices and fruit are a necessity when it comes to cooler weather and watching the changing of the leaves. Store-bought apple cider just doesn't allow for the kind of added flavor and adventure you can have creating this holiday party staple at home. Adding organic pastured egg whites creates creamy foam that adds a rich flavor and protein to this autumnal classic.

Juice pears, apple, ginger. Pour mixture into a saucepan with cinnamon sticks and bring to high heat without boiling the mixture. Reduce heat and simmer for 20 minutes to fully infuse cinnamon spices. Place contents in blender, pour in egg whites slowly, and blend until frothy.

Personal Touch:

PUMPKIN SPICED LATTE

Makes two 16-oz. servings

1 cup of fresh brewed coffee

½ cup full-fat coconut milk

2 dates

1–2 tbsp. pumpkin

$^1/_8$ tsp. fresh chopped ginger

¼ tsp. cinnamon

¼ tsp. cardamom

1 vanilla bean

Thanks to prominent coffee chains, this seasonal favorite has become yet another treat that we can add to a long list of sugar-packed and calorie-rich holiday season guilty pleasures. However, the fundamentals of this drink are a recipe for super health. Pumpkin, being high in fiber and rich in vitamins, is known to support good digestive health and a strong immune system. This at-home recipe transforms a popular junk-food coffee drink into a healthy choice that you can enjoy guilt-free.

Brew a cup of fresh ground coffee. In a blender, combine hot coffee with all ingredients and blend until smooth. Serve in your favorite mug topped with coconut whipped cream and dusted cinnamon and feel good about every sip you take.

Personal Touch:

GREEN FENNEL TEA

Makes two 8-oz. servings (2 quarts fennel water)

2 tsp. crushed fennel seeds

1 tsp. matcha

squeeze of lime (optional)

Green Fennel Tea is a great ally in the fight to "shed a few." With ingredients like green tea that speed up your metabolism, and fennel acting as a natural laxative, you have a combination that is as healthful as it is helpful in combating weight gain.

Add crushed fennel seeds to a tea infuser. Bring 2 quarts of water to a boil. Pour 1–2 cups hot water into tea cup and over matcha. Add lime juice to taste (optional). Let steep for 2 minutes, stir and enjoy.

Personal Touch:

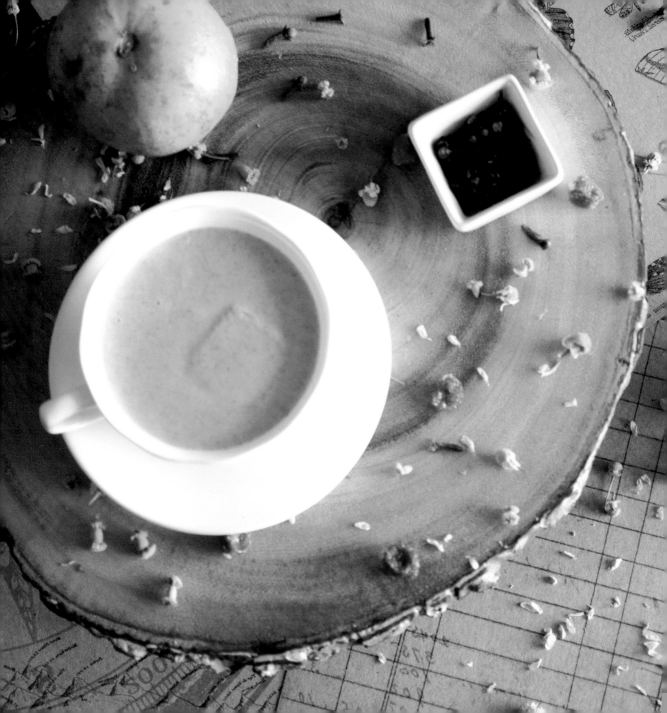

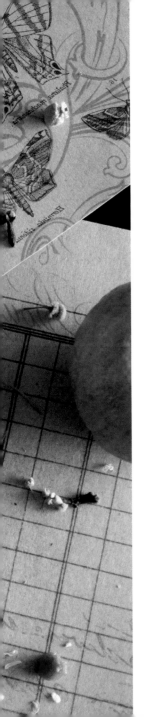

TANGERINE DREAM
Makes one 18-oz. serving

1½ cups chamomile tea

2 tangerines (juiced)

¼ cup almond milk

¼ cup almonds

½ cup dried golden berries (soaked)

1 cup ice

Sweet and smooth, this creamy dreamy goodness will warm up any cool afternoon. Chewy tart golden berries are a great source of protein that delivers a robust and delicious boost to this unique blended tea drink.

Make 1½ cups of chamomile tea. Skin all almonds before blending. Pour tea, milk, and all other ingredients into blender. Blend until smooth. Add tangerine zest. Serve hot or cold.

Personal Touch:

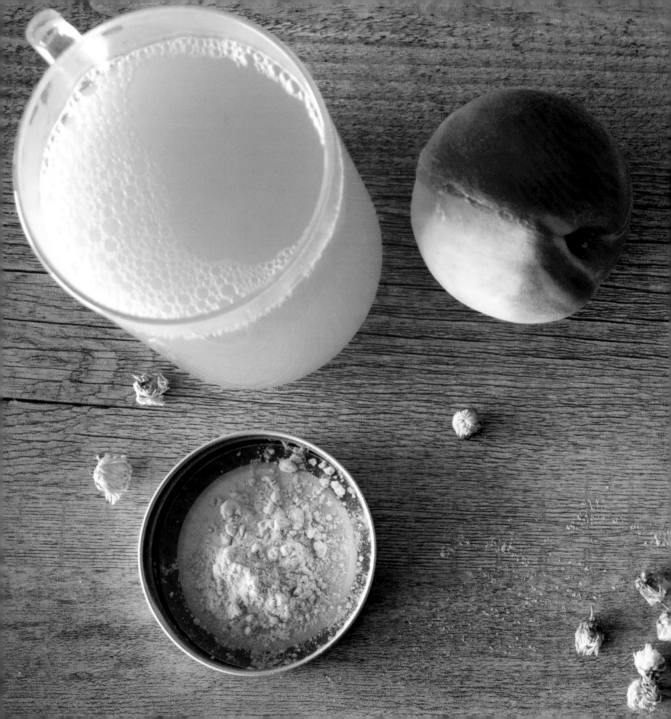

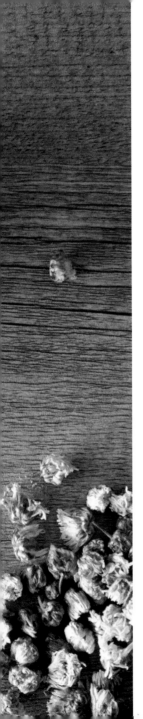

PEACH TEA CIDER

Makes two 12-oz. servings

1 cup apple juice

1 cup chrysanthemum tea

1 cup peach juice

½ lemon (juice)

1 tsp. camu berry powder

thumb of ginger (juice)

3 cinnamon sticks

Here's a super drink that's a surefire way to warm you up and boost your immune system to help you through the flu and cold season. Immune boosters, vitamin C, and great taste are a few things that chrysanthemum tea and camu camu bring to the table to help make this drink the ultimate in illness prevention.

Juice fruit and ginger. Bring a cup of water to boil, pour over an infuser of chrysanthemum tea, and let steep for 2 minutes. In a saucepan, combine juice, tea, and cinnamon sticks. Bring heat up just under a boil, as you don't want the mixture to ever reach a boil. Let simmer for 20 minutes. Pour warm mixture into blender, add camu powder, and blend until smooth.

Personal Touch: _____

_____

_____

SUPER APPLE CIDER

Makes two 8-oz. servings

5 apples

1 orange

1 fennel bulb

¼ cup of mulberries

1 thumb ginger

3 cinnamon sticks

10 cloves

5 cardamom pods

dried peel of 1 orange

This superfood version of a classic apple cider heals the soul as well as the body. Adding a sweet superfood like mulberries brings the added bonus of fighting cancers, bacterial infection, and diabetes to a fall favorite.

Juice apples, orange, and fennel bulb in a juicer. Pour juice and add spices with orange peel into a large saucepan. Heat until just under a boil, as you don't want to boil the mixture. Allow the mixture to simmer for 20 minutes. Pour hot mixture into blender with mulberries and blend until berries are liquid. Serve dusted with cinnamon.

Personal Touch:

DANDELION ROOT COFFEE

Makes two 16-oz. servings

4 cups water

2 tbsp. dandelion root

2 tbsp. chicory root

2 cinnamon sticks

Stevia to taste

This is for those of you looking for a coffee substitute that still has something of that beloved roasted flavor. Bitter dandelion root and spicy chicory double down the intense taste of this healthy coffee alternative without being hard on your digestive system or giving you the caffeine buzz.

In a pot with dandelion root, chicory root, and cinnamon, bring 4 cups of water just under a boil. Let simmer for 5 minutes to release all healing properties. Strain and serve dusted with ground cinnamon.

Personal Touch:

BOOSTERS

These superfood one-shotters can be taken as-is or added to most smoothies to boost the desired effect. Be aware, most have very potent flavor profiles. If taken as shots, you may want an orange slice as a good palate cleanser.

Directions for all Booster recipes

ADD ALL RECIPE INGREDIENTS TO BLENDER.

BLEND ON HIGH UNTIL WELL MIXED.

Energy Boost:

¼ cup coconut water. 1 tsp. wheatgrass powder, 1 tsp. maca powder, 2 tbsp. goji berries, 1 tsp. honey

Brain Boost:

¼ cup yerba mate tea, chilled, 1 tbsp. cacao powder, 1 tsp. maqui berry powder, ½ tsp. cinnamon

Immunity Boost:

¼ cup water, 5 drops oil of oregano, 2 tsp. fresh grated ginger, ½ tsp. camu camu powder, 1 lemon (juiced)

Detox Boost:

¼ cup water. ¼ tsp. chlorella powder, 1 lemon (juiced), 3 drops liquid Stevia, pinch cayenne pepper

Anti-Stress Boost:

½ cup almond milk. 2 tsp. maca powder, 1 tsp. acai berries

Beauty Boost:

¼ cup matcha green tea, chilled, 1 tbsp. coconut milk, ½ tsp. camu camu powder

Protein Boost:

¼ cup raw organic whole milk, 1 tbsp. hemp protein powder, 1 tbsp. chia seeds, ¼ tsp. spirulina

Digestive Boost:

¼ cup aloe vera juice, 1 tbsp. flax seed, 1 tbsp. chia seeds, 1 tbsp. mulberries

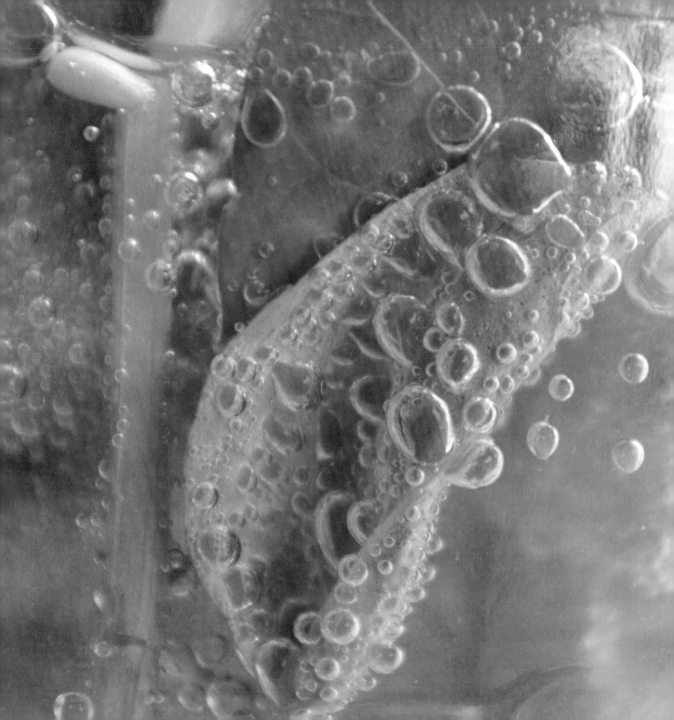

COMMON QUESTIONS

How many superfood drinks should I drink per day?

A loose rule is at least one and no more than 4–5, but it really depends on your goals and what type of superfood drinks you're consuming: smoothies, juices, etc.

Drinks containing very little to no fruit—in other words, mostly vegetables—can be consumed to your heart's content. Juices, especially those with fruit, and other fruit-heavy smoothies should be kept to no more than three because of the excess fruit sugar. Coffees and teas with caffeine should be limited to pre-workout, and for best effect, should not be consumed later in the day so as not to interfere with sleep.

If your goal is weight gain, feel free to consume one before every meal as well as

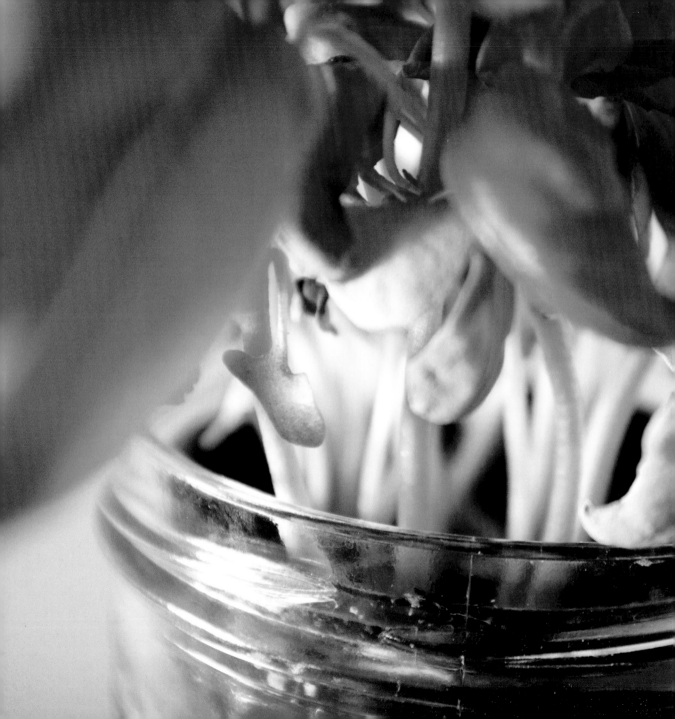

protein-heavy options post-workout. If weight loss is your focus, I would focus on smoothies with minimal fruit and have about 8 ounces before each big meal to satiate and minimize overeating.

What constitutes a "bunch" of greens?

Since we're talking about greens and greens can be consumed with impunity, we can be loose with our quantity measurements. A bunch typically refers to a small head or tied collection of lettuce, or as many leaves as you can hold in one hand. About 3–4 packed cups.

How long do superfood drinks keep?

Fresh is always better and more nutritious, so try to consume what you make within an hour. Keep in mind that certain ingredients can cause the smoothies to thicken tremendously; texture suffers from refrigeration. With that warning:

Smoothies can last up to three days if covered in the refrigerator. Juices, depending on the type of juicer you have, can last covered in the refrigerator for 24–36 hours. Coffees are best consumed right away. Teas can last up to four days in the refrigerator. Infused waters are best consumed within twelve hours; they're so easy, just make a new batch for the day.

Can I freeze superfood drinks or ingredients?

Folks with excess or expiring fruit and vegetables can chop them up and store them in an air-tight bag in the freezer for future use. Freezing superfood drinks is not recommended. If you make too much, just store the excess in the refrigerator for 1–3 days. With juices and some smoothies, excess can be poured into ice cube trays and used in future smoothies.

Aren't alkaloids and oxalic acid in greens dangerous?
In very large quantities and over extended periods of time, yes. However, with a varied diet, this becomes a non-issue.

Alkaloids are chemical compounds found in many foods, including green leafy vegetables. You are probably familiar with some of them already: caffeine in coffee beans and dried tea leaves, morphine from the dried sap of the poppy, and many others besides. They can be toxic in large quantities, but in smaller amounts are actually beneficial. They strengthen the immune system. Consuming the same green in very large amounts day after day can build up the same type of alkaloid in the body, so variety is key.

Oxalic acid, found in many foods like spinach, nuts, seeds, grains, berries, and more, can bind with minerals and have been known to cause kidney stones. Again, this is only a problem when these foods are eaten in very large quantities for months on end.

Vary your diet and drink plenty of water, both of which are inherent when consuming superfood drinks.

I thought raw milk was dangerous?

Not any more dangerous than flying a plane or driving in a car; in fact, it's significantly less. Meat and seafood cause more illness than dairy. And the benefits are worth seeking out milk in its raw form: higher nutritional content, better flavor, you'll be supporting local farmers, and most people previously diagnosed with lactose intolerance no longer suffer symptoms when switching to raw.

Raw eggs?

When consuming raw eggs, you should only use fresh, pasture-raised eggs, preferably from a farmers' market or directly from a local farmer to minimize salmonella. The elderly, young children, and those with weakened immune systems should avoid raw eggs.

It is well documented that raw eggs can prevent the absorption of biotin; however, most of the recipes in this book mix raw eggs with hot coffee or tea, which essentially eliminates that risk at around 160° Fahrenheit.

I just started drinking superfood drinks and I'm bloated and have headaches. Why?

It is important to monitor how your body reacts to certain foods, especially when eating new things. However, most of the time, these are symptoms of detoxing and the stomach reacting to different food combinations. Adding fats with fruit and vegetables, as well as fruit skins, can cause excess gas, so try reducing these quantities until your body can handle them efficiently. You may want to look into taking some probiotics to adjust your gut bacteria.

Headaches can come from an influx of fruit sugar, which you may not be used to, or your body may be flushing toxins. This will dissipate with time as your body washes away the unhealthy while transitioning to your healthier diet.

Do I have to buy organic ingredients?
Organic produce contains more vitamins and minerals than non-organic, so you're getting more for your money. Organic also means significantly fewer chemical pesticides, although some naturally occurring chemicals are still allowed.

There are certain fruits and vegetables that I always buy organic: greens (non-organic crops use large quantities of pesticides) and berries (these can be bought frozen in bulk at a very affordable price). These days, with more and more people concerned with health, organic produce is more prevalent and more affordable than ever before. It's your only body; give it the best fuel you can.

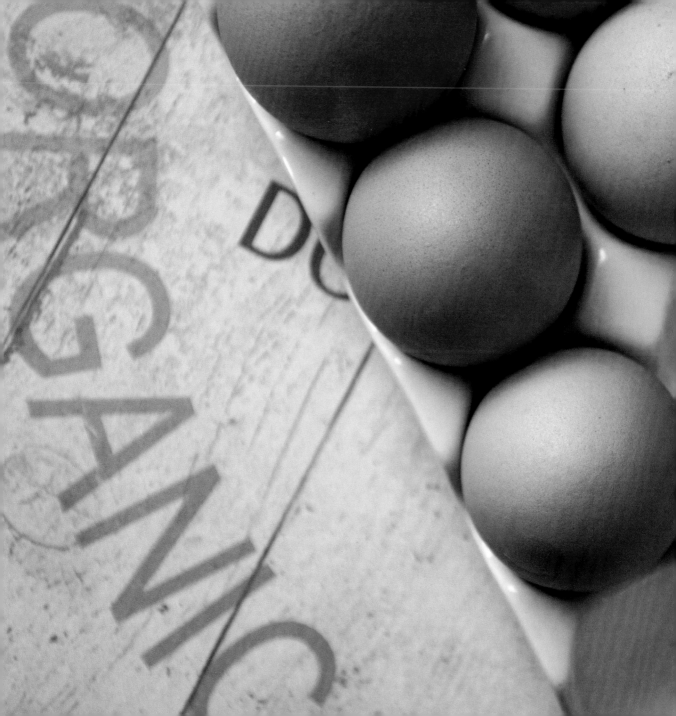

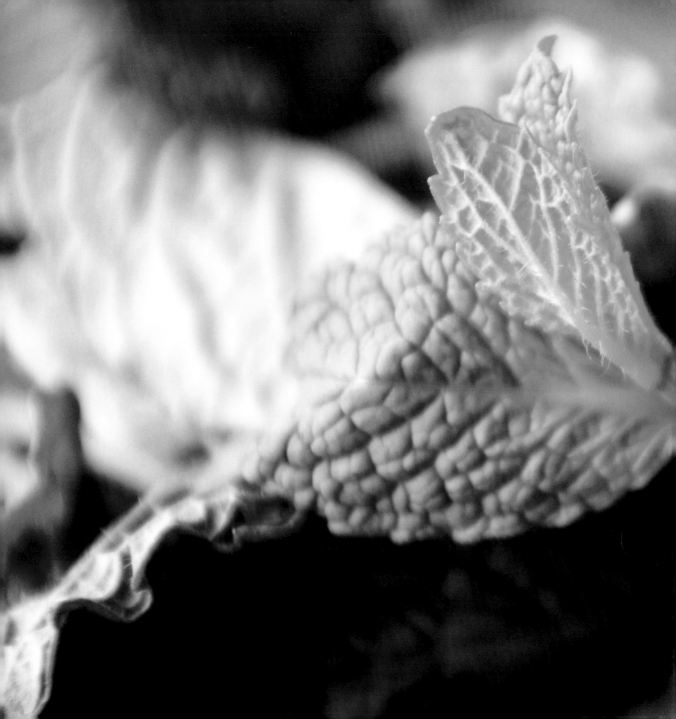

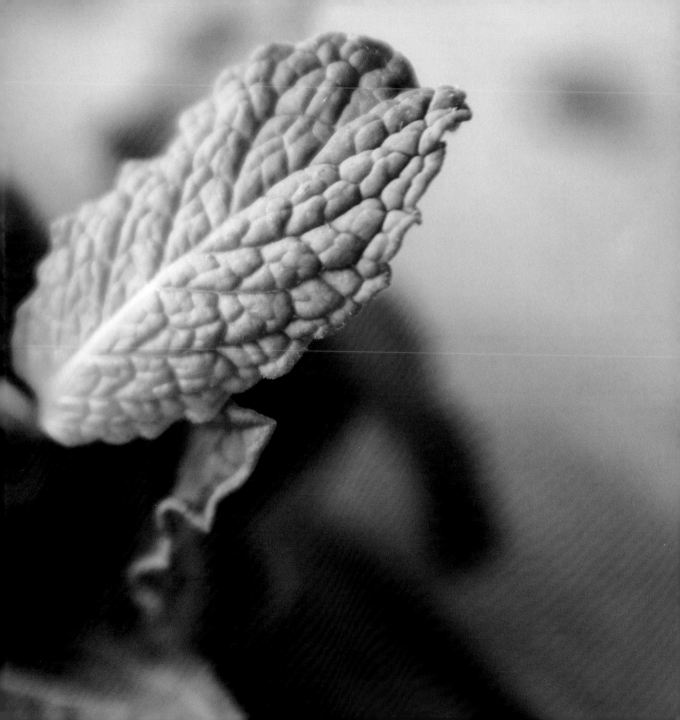

RESOURCES & REFERENCES

Blenders

Vitamix Blender (high-powered): http://superfooddrinkdiet.com/vitamix/

Blendtec Blender (high-powered): http://superfooddrinkdiet.com/blendtec/

Ninja Blender (mid-range): http://superfooddrinkdiet.com/ninja/

Nutri Bullet Blender (mid-range/compact): http://superfooddrinkdiet.com/nutribullet/

Oster Blender (low-end): http://superfooddrinkdiet.com/oster/

Juicers

Breville Juicer (centrifugal): http://superfooddrinkdiet.com/breville/

Omega Juicer (masticating): http://superfooddrinkdiet.com/omega/

Green Star Juicer (triturating): http://superfooddrinkdiet.com/greenstar/

Superfoods

Superfood powders, dried berries, seeds: http://superfooddrinkdiet.com/navitas/

Nutiva Organic Extra-Virgin Coconut Oil: http://superfooddrinkdiet.com/nutiva/

Organic Matcha Green Tea: http://superfooddrinkdiet.com/matcha/

Chlorella: http://superfooddrinkdiet.com/chlorella/

Organic, Fair-Trade Coffee Beans: http://superfooddrinkdiet.com/coffee/

Reading and more...

The pH Myth: http://chriskresser.com/the-ph-myth-part-1

Raw Milk Reality: Is Raw Milk Dangerous?: http://chriskresser.com/raw-milk-reality-is-raw-milk-dangerous

A Prospective Cohort Study of Nut Consumption and the Risk of Gallstone Disease in Men: http://aje.oxfordjournals.org/content/160/10/961.full.pdf

Conjugated linoleic acid in adipose tissue and risk of myocardial infarction: http://www.ncbi.nlm.nih.gov/pubmed/20463040

Local Food Coops: http://www.localharvest.org/food-coops/

USDA National Nutrient Database: http://ndb.nal.usda.gov/

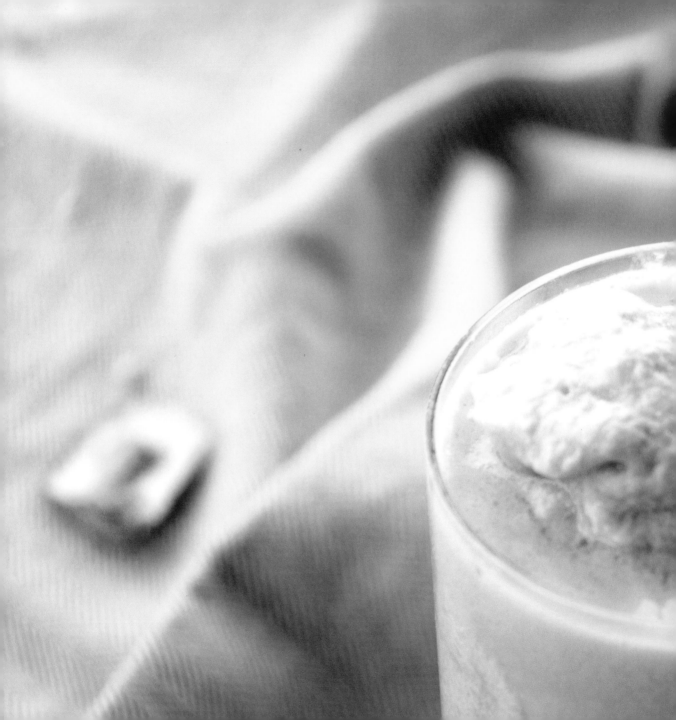

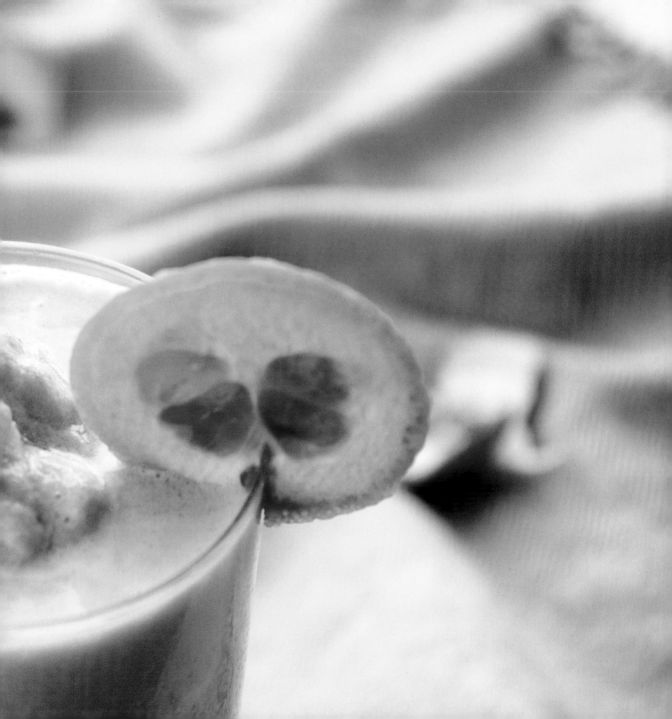

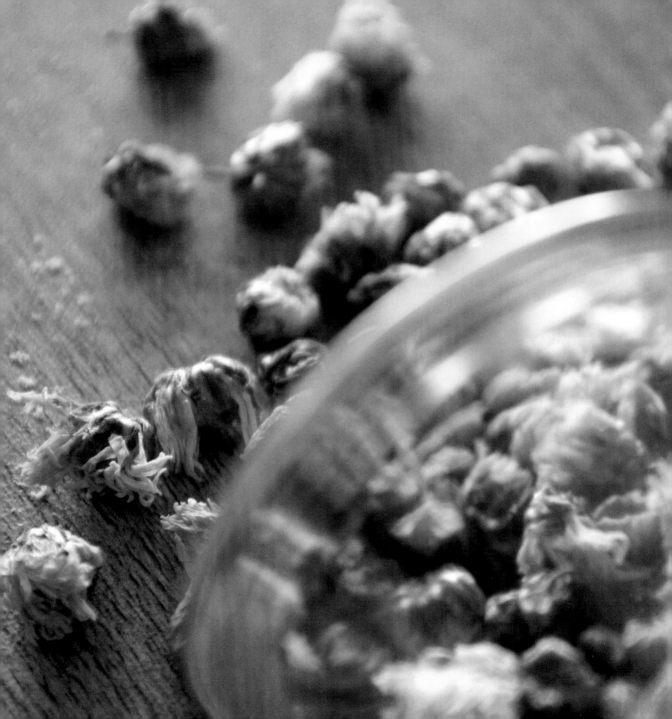

ACKNOWLEDGMENTS

First, a big thank-you to Skyhorse Publishing and everyone whom I've had the pleasure to work with for giving me the opportunity to share, help cultivate, and educate a great deal more people on the topic of health than I otherwise would have been able to reach.

Louise Helton, my unofficial agent, financial advisor, and biggest fan, your love and support is peerless in this world, and I appreciate it dearly.

Eboni, official superfood drink taster, your humor, your pleasant and lively disposition, and your no-holds-barred approach to smoothie photo setup was a necessary addition to the team that we never knew we needed. Thank you.

Leo Quijano II, three-headed lion, master of light, this book would be a dim star amid the firmament of thousands without your brilliant photography. Because of you, it emerges more radiant than the sun itself. Thank you for giving us your Sundays and providing your insight, enthusiasm, and trigger finger.

Adriann Helton, mind-reading graphic stenographer, magnificent arbiter of juice and art, this book would simply not exist without you. Every inch is infused with your gracious input and creative embrace. If the book is a success, it will come as no surprise—everything you touch is left enriched and refined to perfection, including me. If it isn't a success, let's blame Leo.

RECIPE BENEFIT INDEX

INDEX

METRIC AND IMPERIAL CONVERSIONS
(These conversions are rounded for convenience)

Ingredient	Cups/Tablespoons/ Teaspoons	Ounces	Grams/Milliliters
Flour, all-purpose	1 cup/1 tablespoon	4.5 ounces/0.3 ounce	125 grams/8 grams
Flour, whole wheat	1 cup	4 ounces	120 grams
Fruits or veggies, chopped	1 cup	5 to 7 ounces	145 to 200 grams
Honey, maple syrup, or corn syrup	1 tablespoon	.75 ounce	20 grams
Liquids: cream, milk, water, or juice	1 cup	8 fluid ounces	240 milliliters
Oats	1 cup	5.5 ounces	150 grams
Salt	1 teaspoon	0.2 ounces	6 grams
Spices: cinnamon, cloves, ginger, or nutmeg (ground)	1 teaspoon	0.2 ounce	5 milliliters
Sugar, brown, firmly packed	1 cup	7 ounces	200 grams
Sugar, white	1 cup/1 tablespoon	7 ounces/0.5 ounce	200 grams/12.5 grams
Vanilla extract	1 teaspoon	0.2 ounce	4 grams